SOMA

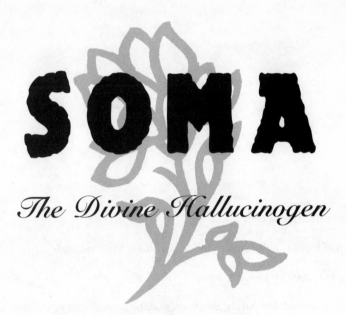

SOMA

The Divine Hallucinogen

DAVID L. SPESS

Park Street Press
Rochester, Vermont

Park Street Press
One Park Street
Rochester, Vermont 05767
www.InnerTraditions.com

Park Street Press is a division of Inner Traditions International

Library of Congress Cataloging-in-Publication Data

Spess, David L.
Soma : the divine hallucinogen / David L. Spess.
p. cm.
Includes bibliographical references and index.
ISBN 0-89281-731-3 (alk. paper)
1. Hallucinogenic drugs and religious experience. 2. Soma. 3. Elixir of life.
4. Alchemy—Religious aspects. I. Title.

BL65.D7 .S64 2000
394.1′4—dc21

99-059445

Printed and bound in the United States

10 9 8 7 6 5 4 3 2 1

Text design and layout by Virginia L. Scott-Bowman
This book was typeset in Times with Mesozoic as a display face

CONTENTS

ACKNOWLEDGMENTS

I would like to thank the following for their support and encouragement during the writing of this book: N. K. B., Katherine Spess, Professor Wendy Doniger, Oscar Ichazo, Mr. and Mrs. Frank Spess, Mr. and Mrs. Edward Reding, Charlie and David Dawson, Kathleen Knoth, the late Professor R. T. Wallis, Dr. Taylor Scott, and Dr. Edward Young.

INTRODUCTION

Throughout history there have been legends of a certain plant, known as the "plant of immortality," that contained the "elixir of life." Many miraculous effects were attributed to the use of this plant. It healed the sick, rejuvenated the aged, and bestowed a direct experience of one's own immortality. The plant that produced the elixir of life was eagerly sought out by many individuals throughout antiquity.

Those few who knew about the original plant of immortality always veiled its identity in secrecy. The method for preparing the elixir from this plant was also a well-kept secret. Because of this secrecy, it has always been assumed that this plant and the effects that it inspired were only legendary; however, it can now be confirmed that both the plant and its unique method of preparation did exist. Fortunately, ancient texts give enough clues about the herb that its identity can now be determined. To the best of my knowledge, no one has rediscovered the secret of the ancient elixir of immortality until now. This book describes for the first time the plant of immortality, the preparation procedures for making the elixir of immortality, and the benefits one can attain through its use.

The idea of an "elixir of immortality" mentioned in Chinese, Greco-Egyptian, Islamic, and European alchemy can be traced back to a plant and drink of Indo-Aryan origin called soma. Soma was a unique psychoactive and visionary elixir. The divine soma drink was said to induce luminous ecstatic states that enhanced paranormal abilities. Consuming the drink induced the experience of inner light, which led to the development of an interior body of light or energy that was coextensive with a subtle universe behind matter. This subtle universe was conceived as the root cause and precursor of our physical universe. It was through the development of this spiritual body of light that humans first gained immortality. The ritual use of the soma drink was believed not only to rapidly aid in the spiritual development of this invisible immortal energy body, but to be the actual origin of the knowledge of such a body's existence.

Herbal drinks like soma were used in what have been called the Mystery Religions. I touch upon some of the mysteries in these religions, and in doing so reveal some of their secrets. I also show that the ritual of the soma ceremony, in which the soma drink is prepared, has influenced the traditions of herbalism, alchemy, magic, theurgy, Neoplatonism, Gnosticism, and Hermeticism.

Ethnobotanically, the implications of the discovery of the elixir of immortality for the development of new herbal drugs, as well as new therapies and methods of spiritual advancement, are enormous. Every indication points to the fact that the elixir of immortality contains compounds that work directly upon consciousness, rapidly eliciting profound experiences of insight and understanding that could otherwise be achieved only through many years of meditation. The implicit fact that paranormal abilities are discussed in the ancient texts, in association with the explicit use of the elixir of immortality, must also be considered in a broader understanding of human consciousness and spiritual development.

1 SOMA AND SACRED HERBALISM IN THE ANCIENT WORLD

Soma is the name of one of the most sacred plants of the ancient world. The drink made from this divine herb was known not only as a panacea but also for its powers of rejuvenation and increasing longevity. Soma also gave its consumer paranormal abilities and a direct experience of immortality. In the written documents that we possess, no other substance predates soma as a candidate for the "alchemical elixir" and "water of life" that later appear in various Western mystical traditions.

Knowledge of the soma drink and the earliest rituals surrounding its preparation were kept secret, and, with the exception of a single text called the Madhu Brāhmaṇa, this knowledge was never written down. We know of the Madhu Brāhmaṇa only by references to it in other texts; no manuscript copy of it exists. The ancient knowledge of soma must then have passed among select groups of priests only in oral traditions. The secret of soma and its preparation, as well as the secret essence of the Vedas themselves, was called the *madhu-vidyā* or "honey doctrine," the oldest references to which are contained in veiled, cryptic religious riddles found in the hymns of the Ṛg Veda, the oldest Indo-European written document. The hymns in this text appear to have been composed mainly in India in the period between 1800 B.C.E. and 900 B.C.E., but it should be pointed out that the ideas, mythology, and cosmology concerning the soma plant and its drink are much older than the dates when these hymns were committed to writing.[1] The priests who wrote the hymns drew upon a vast array of background myths, which in most cases are never fully explained or defined in the text. Thus it has been suggested that many of the Ṛg Vedic myths, much of the cosmology in the hymns, and the soma ceremony itself date back to when the Indo-Iranian peoples were still located in central Asia, sometime around 4000 B.C.E. to 3500 B.C.E.[2]

The mystery and secrecy surrounding soma evoke many unanswered questions. What exactly were the effects attributed to the sacred soma drink in the Ṛg Veda, and why was it considered a miracle drink? Was the soma drink prepared from a single psychoactive and medicinal plant or from a combination of several sacred plants with different psychoactive or medicinal ingredients? Was this soma drink a stimulant, sedative, or divine hallucinogen? Did ancient herbalists have secret knowledge, now unknown to modern science, about a medicinal and psychoactive drink prepared from various herbs that could heal the sick and even bestow paranormal abilities upon the consumer of the beverage?

It seems obvious that herbalists of the ancient world would have discovered many secrets about plants, plant combinations, and dosages over tens of thousands of years of experimentation. The use of such plants in a ritual setting was probably first developed in primitive shamanism, but over time, with the rise of sophisticated civilizations, the rituals and plant combinations would have certainly become more evolved and more precise, reaching far beyond their original shamanic origins. Unfortunately, much of this ancient herbal knowledge has been lost. The uses of these plants and their accompanying rituals, however, can still be glimpsed in ancient archaic languages, mostly in riddle or coded form. The information we do have indicates that many of these sacred plants, when used alone, but especially in combination, had great therapeutic potential for mental and physical healing and included a large array of even more profound effects.

Because of the slow progress of science in isolating and understanding the activities of the compounds in many sacred plants and plant combinations, the mysteries surrounding most of these plants remain intact. This is particularly true when the plants are used in specially designed psychotherapeutic rituals in which their therapeutic effectiveness is significantly enhanced. Only recently has ethnobotanical and pharmacological research begun to uncover these once-secret herbal techniques used for healing, rejuvenation, and the inducement of paranormal effects and the experience of immortality. This interest in ancient herbal rituals, I believe, will eventually create a whole new branch of ethno-psychotherapeutic practices within modern medical science.

The therapeutic effectiveness of the ancient world's use of sacred plants stems from the combination of medicinal compounds that work in a variety of ways upon the physical body with other psychoactive compounds that induce certain types of altered states of consciousness. The results of these combinations can have profound effects on the physical body, altering consciousness so as to induce it to use the body's own healing systems. These ancient medicines, and the model in which they are employed, reach the patient in important ways that allopathic medicine does not. For example, these plants and rituals have been shown to be successful in cases where the remedies of allopathic medicine have been exhausted or the prognosis is terminal. Even modern scientific studies, in what little they have explored of the known sacred plants and their combinations, have determined experimentally that the altered states of consciousness induced by these plants do have the ability to affect and heal a variety of biological systems. Because of their effects, these types of herbal rituals are currently called *hallucinogenic* or *psychedelic medicine*. The ancient soma ceremony is just such a type of medicinal ritual; it uses a sacred plant or plants to heal, rejuvenate, regenerate, induce paranormal affects, and gain a lasting experience of immortality.

Terms like *hallucinogen* and *psychedelic* (meaning "mind manifesting") are often used in both scientific and popular literature to describe plants that affect the nervous system and that are used in many sacred religious rituals for healing, divination, and for inducing altered states of consciousness. These terms, however, are now considered inaccurate for such plants. We have used *hallucinogen* in our title simply because of its familiarity, but we should also emphasize the fact that the use of this term is falling out of favor because its connotations lead to inaccuracies with regard to sacred plant usage in traditional cultures. This inaccuracy is also the case with regard to understanding the effects attributed to soma because most, if not all, of them cannot be strictly classified as *hallucinations*, a term that should now be reserved for certain types of mental illness and psychotic states.

At the turn of the nineteenth century, William James defined various types of hallucinations by saying they are often talked of as mental images projected outward by mistake. But when a hallucination is complete, he argued, it is more than a mental image—it is a strictly sensational form of consciousness, as good and true as if there were a real object there. The object happens not to be there, that is all. James thus distinguished between true hallucinations, which appear objectively real and "fool" the perceiver, and pseudohallucinations, which lack the character of "objective reality." According to this terminology, the hallucinations produced by sacred psychoactive plants in shamanic rituals could be a mixture of true hallucinations, pseudohallucinations, and illusions (perceptual distortions).

James's definitions, however, do not fit well with what the Ṛg Veda says about soma. The soma drink described in the Ṛg Veda produces paranormal effects in the consumer that can neither be considered hallucinations nor be defined by modern neurochemistry. It is in the text of the Ṛg Veda that the earliest examples of miracles produced by human beings rather than gods have been recorded. I shall discuss these miracles in full, shortly.

The question of whether soma was a divine hallucinogen or simply a stimulant or sedative has been hotly debated for decades, but has never been settled because not all of the evidence has been presented. When gathered from the hymns, the evidence points to soma having all three effects. It is certainly a stimulant; by drinking it the priests and their gods are invigorated.[3] It is also shown to have narcotic, sedative, and even debilitating effects when it is overconsumed.[4] In addition, visionary experiences are clearly associated with soma in the Ṛg Veda, and Indian medical books specifically state that the chief means of producing visions is by use of the soma drink. In the Ṛg Veda (8.48.3 and 9.87.9) drinking soma causes the priests to have visions of the gods, and it is through soma that the gods were first discovered.

Whether or not soma induces visionary experiences must depend on how it is prepared in the ceremony. As a drink, it could not always have induced visonary experiences with strong hallucinations because the Ṛg Veda indicates that others in addition to the priests took soma on a daily basis for long periods of time. It would have been not only impractical, but probably impossible, for soma to have been prepared as a hallucinogen in these cases. If soma were always hallucinogenic, it would have interfered with the completion of the soma ceremony itself, which was of paramount importance for maintaining the stability of the cosmos, order, fertility, and life on earth. The soma drink prepared in the ritual must have varied according to the different parts of the ceremony that were being conducted. This leads to the conclusion that the soma drink probably induced states of ecstasy and well-being at certain dosages and that it could also induce visionary states or hallucinations at other dosages or when other plants or plant parts were added to the preparation.

With regard to the light phenomena, out-of-body experiences, the experience of immortality, and other unusual paranormal effects mentioned in the hymns, the soma drink in the Ṛg Veda has all the hallmarks of being a divine visionary drink. The hymns also suggest that these effects may result from soma's being prepared in different ways and in various combinations during the ceremony. There is considerable evidence in the hymns of a variety of soma drinks, made during the ceremony, that produce stimulation, sedative states, and what can popularly be called hallucinations, all of which can be attributed to different forms of soma. The single most important effect that soma induces is a state of divine ecstasy, and it is through this state of ecstasy that paranormal experiences are mediated. This inducement of a state of ecstasy, along with light phenomena and paranormal effects, is what most closely connects soma to a divine hallucinogen, creating what is now called an entheogenic experience.

The word *entheogen* is derived from the Greek word *enthous* or *enthousiasmos*, meaning "divine indwelling" or the "god within one," and an entheogen thus reveals the divinity or deity within a person after it is consumed. I use *entheogen* in place of *hallucinogen* as a more appropriate term for the effects of sacred plants. While the term *psychedelic* can still be used to denote consciousness expansion, *entheogen* is the best term to describe the plants and their by-products used in ritual and sacred contexts. The word itself was coined by Carl A. P. Ruck, R. Gordon Wasson, and others to replace the above-mentioned shortcomings of the terminology of hallucinogen, psychedelic, psychotomimetic, and so on. Wasson offers several definitions of the word *entheogen* as it applies to psychoactive plant use. One is simply that of having an experience of the god within after ingestion of the plant.[5] Another definition is any plant that was and/or is being used in holy agapes and that affords the celebrants what they consider supernatural insights.[6]

The original soma plant, and the various drinks that were prepared from it, along with its accompanying ritual, must be classified as inducing an entheogenic experience in the consumer based upon the descriptions in the Ṛg Veda. The unusual experiences mentioned in association with soma are connected with divine ecstasy, and these experiences are markedly different from hallucinations. Any plant that can induce an ecstatic state that leads to an expansion of consciousness of the divine could, by definition, be called entheogenic. All of the experiences described for soma inebriation in the Ṛg Veda can be attributed to ecstatic states. These ecstasies lead to paranormal activity and healing, which are not associated with mental illusions. Thus the term *hallucination* does not fit the experiences that are attained through the consumption of soma as described in the Ṛg Vedic hymns. The ecstatic experience and its associated miracles are connected more with paranormal activity than with illusions, fantasies, or false impressions. This is not to say that visual imagery, photic experiences, and expansion of consciousness beyond physical-body awareness did not take place, only that because of the effects of the soma drink and soma ceremony these paranormal abilities could occur at any time, even outside of the ritual context. The ingestion of soma facilitated extraordinary events and induced a type of permanent state of being that was retained by a person even beyond the ritual use of the drink. One example of this is the ability to walk on water, which is first mentioned in the Ṛg Veda. In that text a number of soma priests are described as being able to walk on water at any time, and this feat is accomplished by various *somapas* (soma sages) at least nine other times. Many of these *somapas* were considered powerful sorcerers and were called upon numerous times for their unusual abilities. One such group was the Kaṇva clan, who developed the soma ceremony and wrote many of the hymns in the Ṛg Veda.

2

LIGHT, ECSTATIC STATES, AND OTHER EFFECTS OF SOMA

SOMA AND MYSTICAL SOLAR CULTS IN THE ANCIENT WORLD

The ritual use of sacred plants to induce entheogenic experiences was common among certain shamanistic, medicinally oriented, or priestly classes in ancient world cultures. In most cases, the experiences associated with entheogens were connected directly with light and light phenomena. It is not unusual to find sacred entheogenic plants prominently associated with solar cults connected with healing, rejuvenation, and immortality rituals, and this is especially true of the soma plant and drink in the Ṛg Veda.

The soma plant itself and the experiences it brings about are closely associated with light and transference by light to realms beyond our own. The Ṛbhus, a group of ancient soma sacrificers, were said to have entered rays of light, being transfigured into luminous subtle bodies. Through drinking soma they became resplendent with the golden luster of the sun and attained immortality.[1]

The soma plant and the drink prepared from it were used ritually in association with various "operations of the sun," which functioned both on a macrocosmic and microcosmic scale to induce both exterior and interior light phenomena. The consumption of the soma drink helped priests come into contact, through the medium of light, with the deity Soma, experienced as an inner radiant ecstasy. By the internal seeing of the luminous *amṛta*, one was said to gain that *amṛta*. The experience of the abode of Soma, which was a pure realm of light beyond the material universe, was associated with the *madhu-vidyā* honey doctrine, the source of divine knowledge in the Ṛg Veda.

Tradition tells us that sacred plants, including soma, were thought to have unique properties as storehouses of light, an attribute that seems to be associated with the entheogenic effects of these plants. The Gnostic Manichaeans, for example, whose tenets were mainly derived from Indo-Iranian sources, believed that certain herbs and trees were particularly rich in particles of light.[2] The same idea is found in the Ṛg Veda in association with the soma plant and its juice; the plant is said to glow and its juice to be bright in color. Priests such as the Ṛbhus and other *ṛṣis* who drink soma were said to glow, and Indra, the main deity who drinks soma during the ceremony, is called the glowing god. Because of its luminous attributes, soma juice became directly associated with luminosity, brilliance, and the origins of light in the universe.

The beliefs of the Manichaeans were similar to those of the *somapas*. The Manichaeans believed that plants and human bodies contained the greatest number of the captured energetic light particles that were imprisoned in matter at the time of creation. Through the process of ecstasy induced by consuming sacred plants, one could absorb the entheogenic light from them and trigger one's own inner light, with the goal of bringing this light back to its source upon reentering the divine realm of light. This restoration of captured light particles to their original heavenly home of light enabled one to gain immortality. The Manichaeans saw these special sacred plants as important means for obtaining salvation. Chaste and strict vegetarians, the Manichaeans were known to have used entheogenic plants in their religious rituals. It is suspected that their knowledge of such plants originally came from the much older soma ceremonies of the Ṛg Veda, since the procedure of the return of the imprisoned soul of light through the use of sacred "light-inducing" plants is also the central focus of the ancient Ṛg Vedic soma ceremonies.

Soma and Luminous Phenomena

Entheogenic plants are often said to induce light phenomena in association with divine inner experiences. In the Ṛg Veda, soma is described as giving light to all luminous bodies, and the creation of radiant light phenomena plays an important part in the soma ceremony. The hymns associate soma with all light phenomena, whether in the physical universe as starlight, sunlight, moonlight, lightning, fire, and all glowing energies or within human beings as internal, luminous mystical experience. Indeed, soma is said to be the origin of all light phenomena in both the macrocosm and microcosm. It both creates glowing radiance and gives one the experience of light.[3]

In the Ṛg Veda, soma and other plants are said to have a luminous appearance. The types of luminous phenomena, both internal and external, that entheogenic substances produce are usually of white light, golden light, or varicolored or rainbow light. With soma, mention is also made of "clear light," sometimes associated with rain and with certain mystical states of being. In addition, red, white, and gold light are associated with the soma drink, and red, orange, purple, gold, and white light, among others, are associated with soma inebriation. Light phenomena are associated with profound ecstatic states, and they are almost always associated with the ingestion of hallucinogens. It is difficult to see stimulants alone producing these kinds of effects, which gives credence to the view that soma was a divine hallucinogenic plant extract or admixture.

One problem with this view is that from the soma hymns it appears that the experience was mostly internal. It is not clear whether the priest saw white and gold light externally or only internally. If seen only internally, then the experience was based mostly upon the background cosmology, rituals, fasting, and maybe a mild psychotropic trigger. The experience of leaving the physical body that the hymns describe, however, seems more closely related to entheogens. Since the ritual is supposed to lead to immortality and the extension of the pneumatic or subtle body of light, it would seem that entheogenic light-inducing effects are needed.

It is also important to mention that soma ingestion, according to some Ṛg Vedic hymns, can be dangerous, a danger that is also connected with the light phenomena. This suggestion also points to soma being a divine entheogen rather than merely a stimulant. Soma is said to be like a wild bull that is restless, and barriers or fences are put around him internally to hold him in check. If he gets loose, one tries to grab him, but he can slip away and overpower everything. This metaphor more appropriately describes the nature of an entheogen rather than a stimulant or sedative.

Whatever the danger the soma drink could cause, it was not lethal. Although drinking certain soma admixtures can cause one to collapse and fall down, nowhere in the Ṛg Vedic hymns do we find that drinking soma causes death. The real danger of soma, according to the hymns, seems to be more related to its ability to produce visions that are too strong, which again points to its being a visionary entheogen. In the hymns soma is asked, "do not terrify us; do not harm our heart with your brilliant or radiant light." "When we have drunk you soma, be good to our heart." Soma is asked to join closely, like a compassionate friend, so he will not injure us when we drink him.[4]

The internal colors associated with soma as described in the Ṛg Veda are the same colored lights seen in meditation and mystical experiences mentioned in the earliest Upaniṣads.[5] In the soma ceremony these colored lights are associated with the heart-space, which lights up after soma is drunk. The rays seen in deep meditation, according to the Upaniṣads, are seen in the heart as well and are rainbow colored. In the soma ceremony these exact colors are seen in what is called the "heart-sun" after soma is ingested. According to the soma tradition the seat of the soul resides in the heart. These colored rays of the heart-sun are then used as threads during the soma ceremony to weave the inner, pneumatic pillar of light, the immortal soul that extends upward.

The cosmic pillar of light, called *stambha* or *skambha* in Sanskrit, is a fundamental part of the ancient Ṛg Vedic soma-ceremony cosmology.[6] A similar pillar also appears in the Eleusinian Mysteries, in which the sacramental use of an entheogen has also been proposed. There we find that the ceremony was conducted in a darkened chamber or initiation hall resembling a cave, just as in the soma ceremony, where the universe and one's heart are both seen before creation as dark caves. In the Eleusinian Mysteries, participants spoke of the division between sky and earth melting away into an illuminated pillar of light.[7] This cosmic pillar of light is used to separate the heavens from the earth during the creation in order to introduce light into the darkness of chaos, and it is the radiant road by which one can move upward and downward, both out of and back into this world. In the soma ceremony the pillar of light represents the radiant core found within the heart-cave of our essential being. The soma drink and ritual are techniques used to merge the dual processes of the creation of the universe of light and the creation of light within the heart of a person as his or her soul or essential luminous nature.

It appears that the normally concealed central cosmic pillar of light located at the radiant core of both the universe and of our being is a fundamental psychic archetype, since it is found described in several ancient cultures. It becomes visible under specific conditions, such as when our senses and consciousness are absorbed back into the origin of our being. This cosmic pillar, our true nature as self-originating luminosity, is the cosmic Anthropos, also called a pneumatic body of light. Contact with our essential luminous nature in the soma ceremony and the Eleusinian Mysteries was brought about through the use of an entheogen in combination with a specially designed ritual.

The preparation and ingredients of magical and ritual potions used in the Eleusinian Mysteries show exact formulaic correspondences with the Vedic soma ritual. These correspondences cannot be coincidental but must instead indicate that the Greek pattern reflects the ritual drink of the Indo-Iranian religion.[8] It appears that the soma ceremony had a direct influence upon the formulation of the Eleusinian Mysteries. Like the Eleusinian Mysteries, once a person took part in the performance of the soma ceremony and its internal components he or she achieved a permanent immortal experience that lasted an entire lifetime.

ECSTATIC EFFECTS OF SOMA

In the Ṛg Veda the soma drink induces effects that are called *madana*, *madyati*, *made*, or *mada* in Vedic Sanskrit, which can be translated into English as "ecstasy" or "rapturous joy," "inspiration," "heightened awareness," and "exhilaration," respectively.[9] These ecstatic effects were known to bestow holiness and the experience of immortality, moving consciousness into direct contact with the luminous nature of being. This ecstatic effect of soma inebriation appears to have been the mechanism that mediated all other experiences and effects known to have been obtained from the consumption of soma.

The ecstatic experience also gives one the special knowledge and powers of the healer, prophet, poet, and wonderworker. The Ṛg Veda says that soma, when united with the heart, produces the ecstatic vision, an ecstasy that brings expansion beyond this world, a perception of vastness surpassing both heaven and earth.[10] Many hymns describe profound ecstatic states that come about through ingesting soma juice, producing the experience of joy and bliss.[11] In other hymns, soma is referred to as the inspiring drink; soma drinkers say, "Let us drink soma and become ecstatic, let us drink of the ecstasy that is soma"; the gods are said to imbibe ecstasy and the exhilarating nourishment of soma; and priests become like the gods after drinking soma.[12]

Both the bliss induced by soma and soma itself are referred to as *madhu*, nectar, which is the source of the *madhu-vidyā*, or honey doctrine.[13] By drinking soma, the god Indra enters a state of divine ecstasy, and the hymns say that it was in this ecstatic state that Indra created the entire cosmos. The Maruts, who are deities that help Indra, are said to "drink in the ecstasy" of soma. And it is through these deep ecstatic states that the priest, identifying with Indra, leaves his physical body and ascends to the dome of the sky beyond this world.[14]

Although the ecstatic states induced by soma described in the hymn seem to indicate a divine entheogen was used, other parts of the soma ceremony, including ritual combined with the cosmology, legends, myths, and rhythmic chants, also contributed to creating ecstatic states. Rhythmic chanting not only helps to create altered states, but it also guides the ritual in its ultimate purpose. Ecstasy is certainly attained in the soma ceremony, but it is partly derived from the chanting and ritualized cosmological background.

The hymns describing soma illustrate that it created an altered state of consciousness that helped to concentrate the mind and senses to the one-pointedness necessary to achieve the specific goals of the soma ritual, which varied from healing, life extension, paranormal abilities, and the attainment of immortality. Because of the nature of the background cosmology in combination with the entheogen, rituals, and chanting, it is hard to determine just how strong a drink soma really was. Evidence in the Ṛg Veda indicates that the drink varied in strength according to dilution procedures and various soma admixtures, with the admixtures appearing to be the source of soma's divine hallucinogenic nature.

Soma and Paranormal Abilities

Entheogenic substances are known to increase certain types of psychic experiences and this is certainly true for the soma drink.[15] The Ṛg Veda indicates that the structure of the soma ceremony was purposely designed for enhancing psychic abilities, which are mediated by special states of ecstasy. A large number of paranormal feats are described in association with soma in the hymns. Examples of these are the ability to create consciousness-born or psychogenic creations of any object or type; the ability to levitate and walk on water; the ability to leave the physical body and return to it; the power of expansion of the subtle body or consciousness to include the entire universe; and the ability to exist consciously beyond a physical body.[16] Soma is also credited with powers of rejuvenation and life extension as well as the regeneration of various parts of the physical body. Along with its power to renew and even create life, soma is said to be able to sustain that life perpetually as long as one continues to drink it. Thus the Vedic gods maintain their immortality by consuming soma.

The hymns say the nourishing, life-renewing soma bestows new life on the aged and gives long life.[17] To those who have found its hidden light, soma gives magical power, expansion of consciousness, and eternal life: "The worlds expand to him who from before time found light to spread the law of life eternal."[18] By drinking soma, the sages have become immortal.[19] In the Ṛg Veda, Manu, the first man, was given the "god-loved oblation [soma]"[20] and had a long, nearly eternal existence as a result. The priests in the soma ceremony indentify with Manu and eternal life when they proclaim, "I was aforetime Manu, I was Surya, the sun. . . ."[21] Soma is considered the "life-bestower" because it has descended from the "triple height" that is beyond our created universe of matter.[22]

Every time the soma ceremony was conducted both the ceremonial site and those who drank soma were renewed. Soma was described as producing a golden fountain at the center of the ceremonial site, which was said to be the center of the world.[23] This golden fountain at the center is also the cosmic pillar of light formed in the heart of the priest and the original fountain of youth from which the water of life flows. The Ṛg Veda says, "The sage (Soma) the everlasting one, the milk (soma), the hymns unite them (the priests) with him (Soma) in the place of ceremony, which is ever produced anew."[24] This special seat or altar is seen as the earth's highest point, the center of the universe where the cosmic pillar of golden light is formed and where the priest identifies with the luminous soma pillar, the trunk of the cosmic tree. When soma unites the priest to this golden pillar of the creative energy of the universe, he is able to not only rejuvenate the aged but also bring the dead back to life. By the power of soma both gods and humans are able to produce the most unusual paranormal feats.

In the Ṛg Veda, many stories of continuous self-rejuvenation, restoring the aged to perfect youth, and even raising the dead are mentioned. One story tells of the very aged *ṛṣi* Cyavāna who was completely rejuvenated by soma. The sage Kali was also given back the vigor of his youth when old age was coming upon him; the *ṛṣi* Kaksīvat was rejuvenated when he was one hundred winters old, restored to full youth and strength like a new chariot. The sage Vandana was raised from the dead by soma, brought back to life with his youth restored.

The soma sages called Ṛbhus, who became the craftsmen of the gods and are said to be of the celestial race descended from the stars, rather than from the solar or lunar races, became creators and artificers who were able to create material objects by psychogenesis. They are the shapers who build and repair not with their hands but with consciousness. The Ṛg Veda describes how for Indra the Ṛbhus created, with their minds, horses harnessed by a word. The Ṛbhus also fashioned the cup from which the gods drank their soma and were said to have formed a nectar-yielding cow and calf and to have rejuvenated their parents when they had aged.[25]

Indra is said to have rejuvenated the aged sage Bharadvāja by giving him a secret formula associated with soma. Bharadvāja is the sage who revealed the Ayurvedic system of Indian medicine to the sage Suṣruta.

MEDICINAL EFFECTS OF THE SOMA DRINK

The practice of medicine is well established in the Ṛg Veda; in fact, in one of the hymns, 107 plant remedies are mentioned. With the discovery of herbal medicines, a class of herbologists called the Bhisaj used medicinal plants to treat both physical and mental illnesses.[26] Most of the medicines were derived from plant admixtures or individual plants used in conjunction with magical practices.

The Vedic plant world was seen as a sacred and mystical domain within which the soma plant was the king of all plants and the source from which all other plants were derived. This view is based upon the cosmology that is directly connected to the cosmic tree or pillar of light, through which access is gained to the inner workings of nature. The soma plant itself is the cosmic tree and pillar, providing this access by virtue of its psychoactive nature and through its mythologized cosmic characteristics.

The soma drink was considered the most effective of all medicinal preparations. The soma drink was an elixir that worked both psychoactively upon the brain and nervous system to induce an altered state of consciousness as well as medicinally upon the human body to cure it of various diseases.

Both weakness and disease disappear in the physical body immediately after one drinks soma, a unique and divine medicine.[27] Among its benefits, soma is said to heal eye diseases and give clearer sight.[28] It heals the crippled by uniting and knitting their joints back together.[29] It initiates regeneration and replaces dislocated limbs.[30] Soma prolongs one's life span,[31] and it also replenishes one's store of vital strength and gives the ability to beget many children through its aphrodisiacal and virility-enhancing effects.[32] The juice of the soma plant and the soma mixtures were thought to have more magical potency than any other medicinal herb or plant mixtures on the earth.

Immortality

The wondrous virtues of the soma drink do not end with its paranormal, rejuvenating, and medicinal effects; it also gives its consumer immortality. In the hymns of the Ṛg Veda the soma sages speak of the "great purifying" (soma) that places them in that deathless, undecaying world, where the light of heaven shines eternally:

> Flow, soma drops and make me immortal in that realm where dwells the king, Vivasvab's son, that place where is the secret shrine of heaven. That is the place where all waters are young and fresh. Make me immortal in that realm where they move by consciousness alone. Make me immortal in that realm where happiness, joy and felicities combine, and longing wishes are fulfilled.

During the soma ceremony the *somapas* proclaim that they have drunk soma and become immortal; they have attained the light that the gods discovered.

> The glorious soma has given us total freedom beyond the body and has preserved us from disease. Soma has made us shine bright like fire produced by friction, and given us clearer sight. That soma which we have drunk, immortal in himself, hath entered us mortals. Our maladies have lost their strength and vanished: they feared, and passed away into darkness. This soma is now deposited within us. Soma has risen upward in us, exceeding mightily, and we have now come where men prolong their existence.

All of these descriptions show that the priest becomes immortal by identifying with the deity Soma and the cosmic processes governed by soma in the drama of the universe. He is bathed in the light of soma and has expanded his subtle body in a way that results in immortality and freedom. This inner, anthropocosmic body of light is a luminous consciousness that can leave or expand away from the physical body and travel beyond the earth and heaven. This experience is said to reveal one's true immortal nature. The soma sage thus describes the effects of soma drinking as being like violent gusts of wind that lift him upward and out of his body the way fleet-footed horses draw a chariot skyward. "The heavens and earth themselves have not grown equal to one half of me," says the soma sage; he becomes the greatest of the mighty ones and is lifted to the firmament beyond this world. By extension of his pneumatic subtle body of light, internally generated by soma, the soma sage becomes the cosmic Anthropos of light at the center of the universe where the primal laws of creation originate.

Summary

When we review the main physical effects attributed to fresh soma juice and to soma admixtures in the Ṛg Veda, we find that they have a numerous array of medicinal benefits as well as significant psychoactive effects on the central nervous system. The conclusion one could draw from the Ṛg Vedic statements is that soma could be a stimulant or even a strong sedative, but it was also an entheogen that induced both interior and external light phenomena. A fairly large variety of psychoactive and medicinal compounds would be needed for the soma drink to accomplish everything revealed in the hymns. The characteristics that we have mentioned here point to soma's being an entheogen, but of an extraordinary kind that contains medicinal compounds that not only heal, but also rejuvenate, regenerate, and induce ecstatic states and visual and auditory effects.

The hymns indicate that a variety of drinks called by the generic term *soma* were derived from plant juices prepared during the soma ceremony. In addition, the term *soma* had a significant symbolical and mythological meaning associated with light, and it did not refer only to the pressed sap of a single botanical plant but to a divine prototypical plant of heavenly origins that was connected to light phenomena. The evidence in the Ṛg Veda suggests that a number of different soma drinks were prepared during the ritual, which usually lasted a minimum of three days or longer. These drinks could be made from the soma plant alone or from various plant saps (also called soma) added to the pressed-out juice of the soma plant. This would still be in line with the actual meaning of the word *soma*, since "pressed-out sap" could refer to the juice of various plants mixed together to produce the ceremonial drink. This interpretation is also in accord with the idea in the Ṛg Veda that soma is the sap that flows through all plants and that a prototypical plant of heavenly origin gave rise to all plant life on the earth.

Even though we believe that the evidence points to soma being a divine hallucinogen, this need not be the case, as the inducement of ecstasy can be accomplished through a variety of plant compounds that are not considered hallucinogens but have other psychoactive effects upon consciousness. Ecstasy induced by a nonhallucinogenic drink can also lead to the loss of body consciousness that enables a person to enter various altered states, including soul flight. Yet the prominence of soma's association with light phenomena must be carefully considered, because it seems to indicate that ecstasy states induced by at least some of the soma drinks were hallucinogenic. It is only through an exhaustive study of the spiritual aspects of the Ṛg Vedic version of the soma ceremony that an answer to whether soma was a divine hallucinogen can be determined.[33]

3
THE IDENTITY OF PLANTS USED AS SOMA

Although Western interest in soma began more than two hundred years ago, no detailed study of the facts has ever been presented. Even R. Gordon Wasson's research on soma, though very useful, is considered incomplete today. We are in a better position to solve the riddle of the soma plant and soma drinks now than ever before. Both Avestan and Ṛg Vedic studies have progressed since Wasson's landmark book *Soma* was published in 1968. In addition, the study of psychoactive and medicinal plants has advanced significantly. Major botanical breakthroughs on both the Avestan *haoma* plant and the Ṛg Vedic soma now make it possible to draw some conclusions about the identity of the soma plant.[1]

Many researchers who have tried to determine the identity of the soma plant in the Ṛg Veda have relied too heavily upon what the Iranian Avesta says about *haoma*, its counterpart. Even though the *haoma* and soma plants have much in common, it cannot be overstated that the soma of the Ṛg Veda differs in many respects from *haoma*. These differences are the result of non–Indo-European influences upon the composers of the Ṛg Vedic hymns and the subsequent alteration of both the soma ceremony and the plants used in it.

Hardly isolated, the Indian subcontinent had from ancient times established trade contacts with various regions of the world, including central Asia. Artifacts uncovered from the ancient Indus Valley culture of India, which flourished from about 2800 B.C.E. to 1200 B.C.E., show without doubt continuous contact with central Asia and the Aryans at or before 2800 B.C.E.[2] The Indus Valley appears to have been a meeting place for a number of ancient cultures, including that of the central Asian Aryan people.

Because of this ancient contact, the hymns of the Ṛg Veda are a combination of original Aryan conceptions and ancient indigenous Indian elements, mixed with elements from other cultures.

The Ṛg Veda does not speak of any of the large cities of the Indus Valley culture, whose urban phase ended around 1900 B.C.E. It does refer, however, to ruined places where one might collect pots, potsherds, and other objects for ritual purposes. This indicates that those post-invasion Ṛg Vedic hymns were composed after 1900 B.C.E. Archaeological finds indicate that remnants of the Indus culture persisted in some form until 1200 B.C.E. The fact that the composers of the hymns collected objects for ritual purposes indicates their respect for the Indus culture and a probable continuation of similar ritual practices, especially since both cultures had been in contact since at least 2800 B.C.E. The sacred knowledge of the Indus civilization persisted among its indigenous inhabitants, such as the powerful Kaṇva clan, who had a major impact on the soma ceremony and the Ṛg Veda.

The indigenous influences on the composers of the Vedic hymns made the soma drinks and plants they called soma different from those purely proto-Indo-Iranian forms of *haoma* that may have existed in ancient central Asia previous to any contact with India, Iran, or the Near East. There is, however, evidence that the Iranian *haoma* drink became more like its Indian counterpart in Zoroastrian Iran at least by 900 B.C.E., or even much earlier than this. This change came about because of the merging of the ancient botanical knowledge of indigenous India and that of the Aryans before and during the composition of the Ṛg Vedic hymns, which created a variety of drinks using various plants with different modes of preparation that were still called soma in the Ṛg Veda.

The Psychoactivity of Indian *Nymphaea* and *Nelumbo* Plants

Although a number of plants were used in the Ṛg Vedic soma ceremonies, there are two genera of indigenous Indian plants, the *Nymphaea* and the *Nelumbo*, that stand out among the rest as being used to prepare soma drinks in the Ṛg Vedic soma ceremony. *Nymphaea* plants are known as water lilies, while *Nelumbo* plants are the true lotus plants. When the genera are used together in my discussions I sometimes refer to both as lotus plants.

India has the largest variety of naturally occurring water lily and lotus plants of any country in the world. They were once so numerous, in fact, that Sanskrit names were not known for many of them. These plants are also well known for producing naturally occurring varieties, which makes it nearly impossible to name all of the varieties that occurred in ancient India. Some of these plants were certainly known as soma and are actually called soma in Sanskrit texts. Despite what has been stated in various articles and books about the nonentheogenic effects of *Nelumbo* and *Nymphaea* plants, some

Indian varieties of lotus and many water lilies do contain a variety of alkaloids and other compounds that are entheogenic.[3]

Here we can mention only a few studies of the psychoactive aspects of these plants as they pertain to our current subject of soma as a divine hallucinogen. Certain indigenous varieties of Indian *Nymphaea* plants, as well as *Nelumbo* plants, are psychoactive and can be visionary and auditory entheogens when the sap or juice of the plant, and certain other parts, are prepared properly. These two genera can also be shown to have psychoactive properties that match those of soma in the Ṛg Veda.

The compounds found in certain *Nymphaea* species are known to cause excitation, ecstatic states, luminous visionary and auditory hallucinations, narcotic sedation, and other psychoactive effects. The experiences are dependent upon the dosage, preparation, and parts of the plant used. The compounds responsible are found in the flowers, sap, nectar, stems, rhizomes, and possibly the leaves. The flowers of certain *Nymphaea* species have been shown to induce ecstasy states similar to those of the drug 3, 4-methylene-dioxymethamphetamine (MDMA), popularly known as "ecstasy."

In the nineteenth century the botanist de Candolle stated that the sap of lotus plants could be poisonous if taken in large quantities, but in small doses would merely induce hallucinations. De Candolle may have been using the term *lotus* in a generic way to refer to both the *Nelumbo* and *Nymphaea* genera, because the sap found in certain parts of both plants can be hallucinogenic and even poisonous. In the ancient Egyptian medical text known as the Ebers Papyrus, the rhizome of the *Nymphaea* species is described as poisonous, and in Sanskrit the rhizome of some *Nymphaea* species is called *viṣa*, meaning "poison."

The water lilies of the Nile are of the same species as the water lilies of India; modern taxonomic botany has not been able to distinguish morphologically between the Egyptian and Indian *Nymphaea* plants, which indicates that they are conspecific and must have a common origin. That the Ebers Papyrus states that some water lily rhizomes are poisonous is significant. First, it is a known fact that many "poisonous" plants are both renowned medicines and entheogens. Second, the ancient Egyptians were well known for importing plants into their country and cultivating them for food, medicines, and, most importantly, for sacred religious entheogenic rituals and magical herbal healing. The two most sacred Egyptian plants, the papyrus and water lily, were not indigenous to Egypt. There is good evidence that water lilies were brought to the Nile River valley in ancient times, either from tropical Arabia or from areas further east along the trade routes. This important plant first appears in Upper Egypt, associated with the predynastic race who first appeared there and whose origins have recently been shown to derive from the Persian Gulf region, particularly Iran. It is not improbable that the sacred Egyptian water lily was anciently derived from India via the predynastic race of ancient Iran (Elam). It is also known that Indian *Nelumbo* plants were imported into Egypt and cultivated at a much earlier date than was previously thought.

Not only are some *Nymphaea* species psychoactive, but certain Indian *Nelumbo* varieties are as well. *Nelumbo* flowers, nectar, sap, leaves, and rhizomes contain compounds that are stimulating, hypnotic, and narcotic and that can induce trance-ecstasy states as well as visionary experiences. The psychoactive properties of Indian *Nelumbo* species have been known for a long time. Parts of the *Nelumbo* were mixed with tobacco and smoked for their psychoactive effects, which are similar to the effects of such plants as *Cannabis sativa, Hyoscyamus niger, Datura alba, Datura fatuosa, Datura metal,* and *Papaver somniferum.* All of these plants contain strong psychoactive compounds that are narcotic, hypnotic, ecstasy-inducing and can be hallucinogenic.

The evidence found in the Ṛg Vedic hymns clearly indicates that Indra is initially stimulated by drinking soma, but he also exhibits other effects depending on what soma drink he has been offered. These different effects may indicate that soma juice when consumed alone or prepared in special combinations and in low dosages was a stimulant. But the same combinations in moderate dosages were entheogenic, and at higher dosages were narcotic and dangerous. This can be concluded from the hymns themselves, since Indra exhibits all three conditions after drinking soma. These same pharmacological traits are associated with the compounds and preparations for lotus and water-lily plant drinks.

Soma is mentioned in the hymns as being dangerous, but not fatal, when consumed; the latter is probably due to its preparation. The sap from some parts of the *Nelumbo* plant can be dangerous. The rhizomes of a number of *Nelumbo* species are absolutely psychoactive, but not deadly, whereas the sap and rhizomes of most Indian species of *Nymphaea* are strongly psychoactive and deadly if overconsumed. A warning should be sounded here that certain parts of these two genera of plants are extremely dangerous if not properly used. Death can occur within minutes of ingesting certain parts in high dosages, especially the sap in the rhizomes of some *Nymphaea* species.

MEDICINAL PROPERTIES OF INDIAN *NYMPHAEA* AND *NELUMBO* PLANTS

It should be emphasized that for a plant to be even considered as the soma of the Ṛg Veda, it must have more than just psychoactive effects; it must also have the important medicinal properties of healing, rejuvenation, and life-span extension that are specifically attributed to the soma plant in the hymns. Both lotus and water lily plants, used alone and in combination, supply these important attributes. Even though they can be entheogenic at certain dosages, the various plant parts, when prepared properly and to specified dosages, are important medicines used to heal various diseases, to rejuvenate the heart, brain, and skin, and to increase longevity.

Indian lotus and water lily plants are referred to in Indian medical texts as *rasāyaṇa* or longevity herbs. The medicinal effects of these special herbs include the removal of poisons, improved complexion, increased energy and intellect, strength, life extension, and the attainment of divine vision and audition. These last two qualities are directly associated with the important entheogenic properties of both the soma plant and lotus plants.

Lotus plants have long been known in folk medicine for their important longevity-promoting powers, their ability to increase the mental faculties, and their stimulating effects, as well as for their strength-promoting and rejuvenating effects for the weak and ill. They are also well known for producing an elevated ecstatic state of well-being, and they are credited with important medicinal properties in the healing and cure of numerous diseases. In both ancient India and ancient Egypt, lotus plants were used as amulets that signified the divine gift of eternal youth. The lotus has been associated with rejuvenation and longevity more than any other plant in world history; this alone makes it a candidate for the soma plant used in the Ṛg Veda.

The *Nelumbo* has numerous beneficial anti-aging and rejuvenating properties. Various parts of the plant have been shown to have important properties for both the healing and rejuvenation of aged skin and improving the complexion. The *Nelumbo* is also used to treat parasitic eruptions, ringworm, inflammation, and other cutaneous skin ailments. The plant is also effective in neutralizing poisons throughout the body, and it is traditionally used as an antibacterial agent as well as to increase virility, turn gray hair dark again, increase mental alertness, and induce ecstatic states of well-being. It has also been shown to have important antitumoral effects.

The *Nymphaea* species is credited with many of the same properties as the *Nelumbo*. They are used to maintain a glowing complexion and to rejuvenate aged skin, as well as for a number of skin diseases and to prepare various anti-aging medicines. They also possess antitumoral and regenerative properties, enhance virility, and rejuvenate mental abilities by inducing ecstatic states of well-being. Generally, both species of plants are powerful restoratives and rejuvenators of entire body systems; they also increase one's sexual potency and life span, and they have even been shown to regenerate aged or damaged internal organs and improve brain, heart, and central nervous system functions.

LOTUS DRINKS

Although it is not very well known, in ancient India a special ecstasy-inducing entheogenic drink was prepared exclusively from lotus plants. This fact is symbolically mentioned in the Ṛg Vedic hymns and was associated specifically with the ancient soma drink. A variety of lotus drinks, some made only from the flowers and saps of the lotus, others made specifically from the sap of its rhizomes and stems, were prepared, as well as other drinks made from combining different parts of different lotus plants. These lotus drinks were prepared both as non-fermented drinks and as fermented drinks low in alcohol content.

It was common practice in the ancient world to use various entheogenic plants in fermented beverages. The low-alcohol drinks in the hymns of the Ṛg Veda were obtained through the fermentation of soma juice itself or through combinations of other plants added to the soma juice. The lotus drink described in the Ṛg Veda was sometimes fermented, but many times it was only the juice or sap of the plant that was pressed out and drunk directly to induce ecstasy. It should be emphasized that alcoholic infusions are not necessary to obtain the effects from the ingredients used in the soma ceremony. It is not always necessary to extract alcohol-soluble compounds from plants using alcohol. Simple water infusions of either pressed flowers, flower buds, rhizomes, or pressed juice from the rhizomes of lotus plants could supply the alkaloids and other compounds needed to produce euphoric states with both visual and auditory hallucinations.

Both types of drinks, fermented and nonfermented, were offered to Indra, the main deity of the Ṛg Veda. The most important soma drinks prepared from lotus plants in the Ṛg Veda were made from a combination of pressed sap, called soma, and a separately prepared fermented drink. A ritual drink called soma was also made from lotus plants in a procedure that produced a low-alcohol content containing entheogenic compounds. This drink was differentiated from a regular alcoholic drink called *surā* in Sanskrit. Some fermented *surā* drinks mentioned in the hymns produced an intoxicating stupor that was very different from the inebriation of soma and entheogenic soma admixtures. Yet, the same plants were used in many cases to prepare both soma and *surā*, and it was only the preparations and the various plant parts used that differed. *Nelumbo* plants contain specific alkaloids that block certain receptors that cause alcohol-induced stupor, so when these plants are added to a fermented soma drink, the low-alcohol content actually frees alcohol-soluble alkaloids, which in turn increase the entheogenic potency of the drink while decreasing the normal stupor effects of the alcohol.

The fermented lotus admixture had superior effects compared to the unfermented version. The fermented drink, which was known as the *soma amṛta*, or "elixir of immortality," combined the normal effects of the unfermented soma drink with other qualities for an increased entheogenic potency.

The effects of the lotus drink included: (1) virility enhancement; (2) mental stimulation; (3) the inducement of ecstasy; (4) experiences of light; (5) the experience of blissful, rapturous joy and exhilaration; (6) the expansion of consciousness beyond the physical body, the earth, and heaven to the luminous ground of being, the abode of Soma; (7) divine vision and imagery; and (8) the attainment of immortality while still in a physical body through an ontological reorientation of being outside the physical body.

Even at the time of the Buddha, approximately 500 B.C.E., we have textual mention of an ancient drink prepared from the sap of the rhizomes of lotus plants with flowers of certain colors. Since the Buddhists were Brahmanical heretics, they cared little about expounding upon the ancient soma drink of the Ṛg Vedic Brahmans. Soma is never mentioned in any of the oldest Buddhist texts. Yet, at this time the soma of the Ṛg Veda was still very well known. Merely knowing the identity of the soma plant or plants, however, was not enough to recreate the soma experiences described in the Ṛg Vedic ceremony. This is because of the equal or even greater importance associated with the secret ritual preparation that may have already been fully or partly forgotten by that time.

The various ritual procedures for preparing soma were kept secret and only cryptically referred to in the hymns, but the identity of the sacred soma plant or plants was well known among Brahmans and others outside the priesthood. Soma plants collected for soma ceremonies were often stolen for use by non-Brahmans, both because the plants were commercially valuable and many people wanted the health and longevity effects known to be associated with the soma drinks. A plant as sacred as soma would never be forgotten, even by

500 B.C.E., which is only four hundred years after the Ṛg Vedic period. This is especially true in India, a country that traditionally has retained its connection to its ancient beginnings more than any other ancient world culture, which helps to explain why lotus plants are still considered the most sacred plants in India.

The soma drink can be associated with the lotus drink prepared by the early Buddhists. The lotus was the major symbol of the Buddha and was linked by Buddhists to both the elixir of immortality, personified as water, and to fire, which is the same as the dual forces that produce the entheogenic Ṛg Vedic soma drink during the ceremony.

The Buddhist's lotus drink was prepared from the freshly crushed lotus rhizome, and the Buddha allowed it to be consumed by the monks during certain times, whereas alcoholic drinks were strictly forbidden. Like fresh soma juice, the lotus-root drink is specifically noted to have effects different from those of alcohol. The lotus-root drink was allowed because of its psychomental, invigorating, and restorative effects. The drink provided a calming, brain-stimulating effect that increased the heart rate. Its overall effects would have included invigoration, euphoria, a feeling of well-being, mental acuity, and ecstasy. The Buddha allowed monks to consume the lotus-root drink because it aided their practice of relaxation, concentration, and meditation. Only through overindulgence, either with or without the specially fermented lotus drink of the Ṛg Vedic soma ceremony, would the results go beyond pure ecstasy and healing to hallucinogenic and narcotic effects. The Buddha allowed the consumption of this drink, made from the most sacred plants of India, only during times of food shortages. Once this had passed, the consumption of the lotus-root drink, as well as all parts of the sacred lotus plants, was strictly forbidden.

An important point to emphasize is that both *Nelumbo* and *Nymphaea* plants were extremely scarce, if not impossible to find, on the plains of India during the time of the Buddha. They had become scarce through overconsumption, just like the soma plant. Both plants could be procured only from the mountainous lakes and rivers of Kashmir, where the soma ceremonies were thought to have originated. By 500 B.C.E. these lands were controlled by non-Brahmanical tribes who sold these plants to Brahmans on the plains, which shows that in the time close to the end of the Ṛg Vedic period, after the priesthoods had moved down into the plains, and with the emerging Brāhmaṇa textual literature, certain lotus plants used in the ceremonies were not easy to obtain locally but had to be imported from the mountainous regions in the northwest. This does not mean that previously they did not grow in the rivers and lakes on the plains, just that over time the lotus plants were used by large numbers of separate Aryan clans—and even individuals, according to the Ṛg Veda—who performed soma ceremonies daily. This scarcity also coincides with the drying up of the Saravastī River, which was a major site for soma ceremonies in the Ṛg Veda and an abundant source for lotus plants of all types. It also corresponds to the Brahmanic priesthood moving further east and south from northwest India away from the Indus River, described in the Ṛg Veda as a source of various lotus plants used in the early soma ceremonies. Neither plant grows just anywhere, and overuse could have easily depleted them at various ritual sites.

Furthermore, the parts of these plants that are used ritually contain important compounds that oxidize readily and lose their potency. These parts must be used fresh after picking to obtain some of the experiences described as soma inebriation. This is probably one reason why all ancient soma ceremonies in the Ṛg Veda were conducted along rivers and lakes. Lack of supply, cost, and low psychoactivity may be very good reasons why substitutes were introduced in the Brāhmaṇas for soma plants once used in the Ṛg Veda. Because the Brahmans did not want to cause the extinction of their most sacred plant, they established rules on the use of the lotus, cultivating it on the plains mainly in temple pools where it was generally forbidden to be touched.

The writers of the Brāhmaṇas, who came from the same priestly families as those who wrote the Ṛg Vedic hymns, knew the exact identity of the original soma plant described in the Ṛg Veda. When the real soma plant or plants could not be obtained, or were obtained and stolen—since there was such a demand for the plants—it would have become easier to find substitute plants in order to continue the ritual that was so important for the stability of the cosmos. And so we find in the Brāhmaṇas, which first appear around 900 B.C.E., about the same time as the end of the Ṛg Vedic period, the introduction of soma plant substitutes. These substitutes were introduced when the original soma plant became unavailable to carry on the tradition. At this same time, the ceremony itself became more ritualized and overshadowed the entheogenic experience at its core.

Nymphaea and *Nelumbo* Plants in the Ṛg Vedic Soma Ceremony

Concerning the lotus plant's role in the soma ceremony, it is relevant to mention that in the Ṛg Veda flowers are mentioned as part of the soma drink. An epithet for soma is the word *andhas*, which is related to the Greek word *anthos*, meaning flower. The word *andhas,* also meaning flower, is frequently associated in the Ṛg Veda with *madhu*, the sweet psychoactive nectar prepared from flowers.[4] The word *andhas* can also mean the soma sap, or the nectar extracted from the flower of the soma plant. It is not clear, however, whether it is newly pressed soma sap or an admixture that is referred to as soma.[5] *Andhas* is found almost exclusively in the Ṛg Veda. The word does not occur in the Iranian Avesta, occurs only twice in the Atharva Veda, and is mentioned very seldom in later Indian literature. This word seems to have been selected to convey a specific meaning for the soma plant and its juice, and it indicates that at least part of the soma drink was derived from flowers.

In addition to the soma plant, the only other plants that are frequently mentioned in the Ṛg Veda are various lotus plants.[6] The lotus flower is actually one of the few flowers even discussed in the Ṛg Veda.[7] In Vedic Sanskrit the word *puṣpa* means "flower" and the term *puṣpavati* is used in Ṛg Veda 10.97.3. One name for the lotus is *puṣkara*, which means "nourishing" and is derived from the same root as *puṣpa*. The nourishing quality of these plants relates to their restorative and rejuvenating effects as well as to special psychic states and feelings of well-being and ecstasy.

In the Ṛg Veda soma was also considered a food in and of itself, and lotus plants have an ancient history as a restorative and rejuvenating food.[8]

Lotus and water lily plants are referred to not only by certain names in the Ṛg Veda but also by their growth patterns or plant parts. It should be kept in mind that the names do not refer to the whole plant, but just to the parts or effects of some of these plants. Lotus plants, more than any other Ṛg Vedic plants, were seen as combining a number of plants into one because of their unusual growth patterns. Each of their parts including flowers, flower parts, nectar, stems, rhizomes, and sap must have had different names.

These names often refer to only one part, such as the flower, or to one of the effects of the plant. Therefore the complete names, or real names, of the lotus and water lily plants known during the Ṛg Vedic period, of which there were a large number of species and varieties, are not mentioned in the Ṛg Veda, and they could easily be referred to by the generic term *soma*, as was the pressed sap of these plants.

The two names used in the Ṛg Veda for water lily and lotus plants are *puṣkara* and *puṇdarika*, but these refer only to an effect and a color, respectively. So what about all the other lotus plants and parts of lotus plants? These must have been called something else, very possibly the generic word *soma*. *Puṇdarika*, which occurs only once in the Ṛg Veda, is used in reference to the white flower of a single *Nelumbo* plant; it refers neither to the whole plant nor to any other part of that plant, nor to any other *Nelumbo* variety. The term most frequently encountered is *puṣkara*. It has been a subject of considerable debate among Indian ethnobotantists whether *puṣkara* refers to a *Nelumbo* or *Nymphaea* plant; in most cases it actually refers to the *Nymphaea* water lily, but not always.

In the Atharva Veda, a text containing ideas and doctrines as old as the Ṛg Veda and including many of the same cosmological views on soma and the soma ceremony, lotus and water lily plants are mentioned by various names that again refer only to parts or attributes of the plants and never to the whole plant itself. Again, this indicates that the whole plant of certain water lilies and lotuses may have been known by another name, such as soma, which referred both to the pressed-out juice of these plants and to the lotus plants themselves.

4 THE AŚVINS AND THE ELIXIR OF IMMORTALITY

One neglected yet very significant area of research on the Ṛg Veda concerns the identity and role played by the twin Aśvins in both early and later soma ceremonies. The Aśvins' role in the soma ceremony is fundamental and is connected to the preparation of a special soma drink that was considered the "divine soma mead" and "elixir of immortality." There is also extensive evidence that this *madhu*, or sweet mead drink, of the Aśvins was a type of low-alcohol fermented mixture made from parts of plants that contained soma (pressed plant sap) and was therefore considered to be soma itself. There is ample proof that it was the legendary Aśvins' soma drink, prepared during the Ṛg Vedic soma ceremony, that was the origin of all the "elixir theories" later found in many forms of alchemy throughout the world.

Just who and what were the Aśvins? The Aśvins are the twin

physicians of the gods in the Ṛg Veda, and they are associated with fertility and the sun. Athough they are associated specifically with horses, an animal connected with the Indo-Europeans, the Aśvins may not be purely Indo-European in origin. A conception akin to the Aśvins already appears in association with the Indus Valley cultures of India. Whether this association was through central Asian, indigenous, or other external influences is not clear. It may be that the Aśvins, being twins and representing dual principles found in nature, such as fire and water, are related to similar dual motifs found in other cultures. Generally, wherever the Aśvins or Indo-European twin deities appear in literature, they are associated with herbal medicine and the indigenous flora of a region.

In the Ṛg Veda the Aśvins, although associated with healing and the use of many medicinal and poisonous plants, are primarily connected to two genera of plants. These are lotus plants, specifically of the *Nelumbo* variety, but primarily the *Nymphaea* species. *Nelumbo* varieties are true lotus plants, whereas the *Nymphaea* are water lilies. Historically, the Latin word *lotus* has been popularly applied to both genera. One of the most important additives to soma juice came directly from parts of *Nymphaea* and *Nelumbo* plants, which were prepared by the Aśvins during the soma ceremony. It is probable, therefore, that both genera were associated directly with soma as the sap in these plants and through various soma admixtures.

The soma ceremony is a special ritual of herbal mysticism used for healing and attaining various spiritual states, aided in part by a consciousness-expanding entheogenic drink. The lotus plants were naturally used as food sources and medicines and for important religious rites. The *Nelumbo* and *Nymphaea* plants were perceived as different from other plants. Their unusual growth patterns made them seem to be alive, and they had mysterious, even supernatural, ways of growing and reproducing that were connected directly with the sun and moon. Their psychoactive, healing, and rejuvenating abilities further added to their mystique. It would thus seem appropriate for them to be incorporated into a detailed cosmological system. Many of the main deities in the soma ceremony, and of course the deity Soma himself, are directly connected to plant life. Indra, Agni, Soma, as well as the twin Aśvins are connected to lotus flowers in Vedic literature, and even the demons *(asuras)* in the Ṛg Veda have a botanical role.

The Role of the Aśvins in the Ṛg Vedic Soma Ceremony

In the Ṛg Vedic soma ceremonies, the priests drink and also offer to the deities both pure, freshly pressed soma juice and mixtures of freshly pressed soma juice and other ingredients. A variety of drinks are called soma in the hymns, and some of the epithets for soma, such as *madhu* (sweet nectar), refer directly to the ones associated with the Aśvins.

The Aśvins normally prepare medicinal and psychoactive drinks during the soma ceremony. It is their drink that helps make the bitter-tasting, freshly pressed soma juice sweet and entheogenic at all three soma pressings, that is, at dawn, midday, and dusk. The Aśvins' soma drink is ritually mixed with freshly pressed soma juice three times a day to produce the most important of the soma drinks used in the ceremony.

The Ṛg Veda says that soma freshly pressed with stones belongs to the Aśvins.[1] This shows that freshly pressed soma was directly mixed with the Aśvins' special *madhu* soma mixture. Since the Ṛg Veda says that the Aśvins are *madhu*, and that their chariot is made of *madhu*, then when the Aśvins are said to drink soma this means that the priests at the ceremony who are the protégés of the Aśvins are using the plants that the Aśvins represent to form a soma mixture, a soma *madhu* drink. This is one reason soma is called *madhu* or sweet nectar. In many cases, the hymns are actually referring to the soma drink as the Aśvins' soma admixture. The soma juice and the Aśvins' drink are mixed at the ceremony as soon as the Aśvins arrive in their chariot, which is at dawn just before the sun appears. The Aśvins' drink is then added at each soma pressing.

The Aśvins' association with *madhu* is a major divergence between the old Iranian Avesta and the Ṛg Veda. In the old Avesta, *madhu*, as either honey or flower nectar, occurs very rarely. Yet this is a key component in understanding the soma plant and soma drinks prepared in the Ṛg Veda, as well as in understanding the source of ecstasy and the making of the elixir of immortality in the soma ceremony.

In Sanskrit the word *aśvin*, derived from *aśva* (horse), means literally "possessed of horses" or "horse-headed." The motif of horse-headedness and the Aśvins' association with horses has an important botanical significance. The poets of the Ṛg Veda use it metaphorically in the hymns.

The significance of the Aśvins' soma drink is even more important when we realize that they are the divine physicians of the gods. As medical deities, they are themselves forever young and are forever renewed and rejuvenated by their soma drink. They are described in the hymns as continually drinking their soma mixture aboard their chariot yet never becoming intoxicated; their *madhu* soma drink induced ecstatic states and brought about healing, rejuvenation, longevity, and entheogenic experiences rather than intoxication. Eternal youth is another attribute of the Aśvins' special soma drink, and they bring the aged back to youthfulness with their drink in special magical rituals. They even aid the gods when they become unable to help or cure themselves of unusual illnesses or other strange misfortunes.

The Aśvins are mentioned throughout the Ṛg Veda in hymns that are associated with miraculous healings through the use of herbs and magical practices, and they are directly invoked for their healing powers by the Vedic priests who are their protégés. They are always mentioned in twin or dual form, probably because they represent the separation and union of opposite forces, especially in magical healing, rejuvenation, and immortality rituals, as well as in the mixing of herbal preparations at which they are adept. The Vedic priests are the ones who, through the Aśvins' guidance and through supernatural communion with them, have taught the priests the secret herbal formulas and preparation procedures of the various lotus plants.

The Aśvins are said to be lotus-crowned *(puṣkara-srajau)* in both the Ṛg Veda and the Atharva Veda, the two oldest books on the soma ceremony.[2] The same Atharva Vedic hymn that mentions the Aśvins crowned by lotuses says that two great forces have come together, like fire and water or Agni and Soma, through the power of the Aśvins. This entheogenic power enables the priest to generate an interior, glowing body of light like that of the deity Soma. This inner, glowing body of splendor is the same as the *aja-ekapāda-skambha* pillar or trunk of the tree of light that the priest identifies himself with through the agency of the entheogenic drink.

THE AŚVINS AND *NYMPHAEA* AND *NELUMBO* FLOWERS

The Aśvins are directly associated with water, and in several Ṛg Vedic verses they are said to be water born *(abhijan)*, like the lotus flowers.[3] In later literature the Aśvins are associated with the *yakṣas*, water deities that are themselves directly associated with the lotus plant and lotus flowers.[4] The Aśvins are also said to be sons of the submarine fire, which connects them to the same birth source as the dual principles of fire and water, or Agni and Soma. In the Ṛg Veda the Aśvins are said to have the waters as their mother,[5] and they are called "sons of the waters," connecting them directly with water and the medicines that reside in aquatic plants.[6] The Aśvins are also associated with the dawn, which is when lotus flowers open to reveal the golden sun within, and dawn is when they first appear in the soma ceremony. All of these attributes link the Aśvins to the *Nymphaea* and *Nelumbo* plants.

Several levels of meaning can be ascribed to the twin Aśvins, one of which frames them as botanical deities. In the Ṛg Veda the Aśvins are the only deities that are crowned with lotus flowers *(puṣkara-srajau).* While *puṣkara* usually means water lily *(Nymphaea),* in some instances it can also mean lotus *(Nelumbo).* This may depend on the effects of the drink prepared and whether it is mainly entheogenic or medicinal. As far as the Aśvins are concerned, we can say that they are connected to both plant genera, and their soma (pressed plant sap) mixtures are prepared from both *Nymphaea* and *Nelumbo* plants.

The lotus or *puṣkara* on top of their heads symbolizes the star-shaped flowers of specific *Nymphaea* plants. The Aśvins are said sometimes to be horse-headed, and their sun chariot is pulled by horses through the waters of the blue sky. Horses in both the Ṛg Veda and the Avesta are associated with water, and both the heads and hoofs of horses are connected directly to the *Nymphaea* species of aquatic plants in the Ṛg Veda. The Aśvins ride in a supernatural chariot that is said to travel at the speed of thought. The Aśvins' horses are *Nymphaea* flower buds, while their chariot is associated with both *Nymphaea* and *Nelumbo* flowers. It is in the center of their *madhu* flower chariot that they mix the *Nelumbo* and *Nymphaea* flowers together. Their chariot is said to overflow with divine nectar from the ritual mixing of these flowers (Fig. 1).

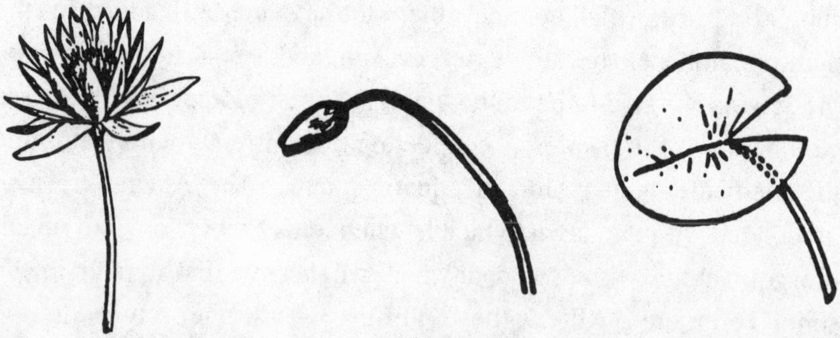

Figure 1. The *Nymphaea* flower and bud associated with the Aśvins' head, and the *Nymphaea* leaf associated with the Aśvins' horses hooves.

Other Ṛg Vedic hymns indicate that the Aśvins are actually the lotus that grows in the waters of the Sarasvatī River, indicating that they are associated with the flowers of *Nelumbo* and *Nymphaea.* Both plants must have grown abundantly in that river before it dried up, for along the northern banks of the sacred Sarasvatī is the location of the largest number of soma ceremonies performed in the Ṛg Veda.[7]

In the hymns, sweet nectar *(madhu)* as soma is directly associated with the Aśvins, and they are asked to come and drink the *madhu* since they are said to be used to drinking it.[8] Here *madhu* means the special soma *madhu* drink of immortality. The Aśvins are said to shine and glow from the imbibing of their special drink, which rejuvenates aged skin and restores youth, and their bodies shine and are described as golden in color, like the color of the soma *madhu.*[9] This is because the Aśvins are actually the lotus flowers that the *madhu* drink is made of. The Aśvins thus are sometimes referred to by the drink that they represent, that is, the ingredients used to make the soma *madhu* drink prepared for them at the soma ceremony by the priests.

There is further evidence in the Ṛg Veda that the miracle-working twin Aśvins are the lotus flowers themselves. As flowers the Aśvins are said to provide the nectar for bees to make honey, and they are associated with honeybees and bee culture in certain hymns where they are said to give *madhu* or nectar to the bees to make honey, which would indicate that they are the flowers.[10] RV 10.40.6 says, "The bee has carried in its mouth the [*madhu*] or nectar from you [Aśvins]." The Aśvins themselves are likened to bees that collect the psychoactive nectar from the golden chambers in the center of the lotus flower, which also represents the sun. The protégés of the Aśvins, who collect the nectar-containing parts of lotus flowers that they then press or mix together to make soma *madhu* during the ceremony, are also likened to bees. This is why the secret of the soma ceremony is called "the honey doctrine." The dual Aśvins are also described as two bees who create *madhu* in the udder of the cow, which represents the sun that dispenses soma sap or milk as *madhu* to the priests. The soma sap is referred to as milk because it is actually milky white before the ingredients the Aśvins represent, which make it golden colored and the elixir of immortality, are added. The sun is the golden seedpod, or the golden nectar chamber in the center of the *Nelumbo* lotus flower, which represents the center of the celestial chariot of the Aśvins.

The Aśvins' Horses and **Nymphaea** *Plants*

The lotus-crowned, horse-headed Aśvins appear before dawn in a carriage drawn by horses or swans. Their horse-headedness is a botanical metaphor: the unopened flower buds of *Nymphaea* sometimes rise above the water and droop downward, resembling a horse's head. Their long stems and drooping buds can resemble swans as well, hence the occasional reference to the Aśvins' chariot being drawn by swans.[11] It is not unusual for some Indian deities, such as Aditi, to have the head of a lotus flower in place of a human head, and this is also the case with the twin Aśvins, whose heads are *Nymphaea* flowers.

The Aśvins' flower chariot is also pulled by horses, which are composed of parts of *Nymphaea* plants. In addition to *Nymphaea* flowers having horse-headed flower buds, they have leaves that resemble the hooves of a horse. In the growth of the *Nymphaea* it is not unusual to see a horse-headed stem rising above four hoof-shaped leaves, two in front and two in back (Fig. 2).

In the later Vedic literature, such as the Taittirīya Saṃhitā 2.3.12.2, horses are said to be born of water, and in the churning of the ocean myth, which can be shown to be derived from the ritual preparations of the Ṛg Vedic soma ceremony, a white horse is produced. White-horse symbolism is closely connected to the lotus plants used in the soma ceremony. The imprint of the hoof of a white horse is used in the construction of the fire altar at soma ceremonies. Agni (fire), the first god to be generated at the ceremony, is born in the water directly from a *puṣkara*, or hoof-shaped *Nymphaea* leaf. In the Ṛg Veda the sun is a horse, as is Soma, and all are symbolically derived from lotus plants.[12] The sun is born of water just as the lotus

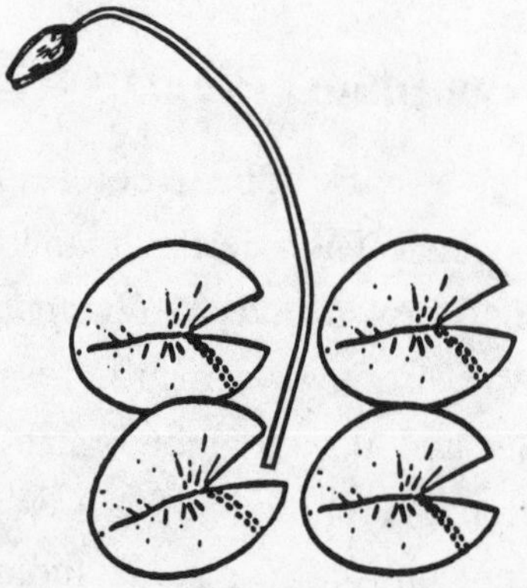

Figure 2. A single *Nymphaea* horse of the Aśvins, showing how the horses of the Aśvins are composed of parts of *Nymphaea* leaves, stems, and buds.

plant. Horse symbolism is generally connected to most deities in the Ṛg Veda because all were associated with the waters of creation. Varuṇa is king of the waters. Varuṇa had a son named Puṣkara, the name applied directly to *Nymphaea* plants. The *yakṣas*, who are the attendants of Varuṇa, are entheogenically seen elflike creatures who have pointed ears and live in another dimension, not ours. The water world is symbolic of this other entheogenic dimension. The *yakṣas* are said to drink strong psychoactive drinks derived from lotus plants, and the Aśvins are called *yakṣas* in the Mahābhārata. Both Varuṇa and the Aśvins are associated with horse symbolism.

In Zoroastrian literature, the deity Apām-napāt is the primal waters of creation, waters also found in the Ṛg Veda and associated with the celestial waters where Varuṇa resides. The Vedic Apām-napāt is called the urger-on of horses. The Avestan Apām-napāt's epithet is "having swift horses." In both the Ṛg Veda and Avesta the horse is a symbol of the water god. In Avestan mythology, the rain god Tistrya takes the shape of a horse and the river goddess, Aredvi, drives four horses. In India, Agni is associated in literature and cult with the horse. This is probably through Agni's identification with Apām-napāt; both Soma and Agni are born from the waters. Agni as a horse and son of the waters is created from the lotus plant in the womb of the waters. This clearly shows a connection between Agni and Soma and lotus plants.

Water lilies that have psychoactive flowers, sap, and rhizomes are especially connected to horses in ancient Indian literature. The Sanskrit *kuvalya* means water lily and is directly connected to the horse of Kuvalayaśva in the Mārkaṇḍeya Purāṇa.

The horses of the Aśvins are said to be varicolored and radiant in the Ṛg Veda.[13] The colors of the horses of the Aśvins connects them to the varicolored flowers of the many indigenous Indian *Nymphaea* species, and they are described specifically as adorning the soma sacrifice,[14] which refers to their being used in a soma admixture. It is clear in the hymns that the flower buds or horses' heads were used in the mixtures made by the Aśvins when they are said to whip or whip up their horses.

When the hymns state that the waters are full of horses, they are referring to aquatic plants of the *Nymphaea* and possibly *Nelumbo* genera. One hymn refers to the Indus, called the Sindhu River, as being rich in horses, chariots, and robes, the robes here being the lotus plants that cover the surface of the water as they sometimes do.[15] The horses are lotus buds and leaves, and the chariots are open lotus flowers. Each lotus flower is rich in nectar, and many hymns note that the waters have covered themselves with raiment rich in sweets, which would be the psychoactive nectar in the flowers themselves. One hymn says, "Herbs rich in soma, rich in horses, in nourishments, in strengthening power—All these have I provided here, that this man may be whole again."[16] This verse again associates soma with horses and is further evidence that the soma plant was associated with *Nymphaea* in the Ṛg Veda.

The Aśvins' Entheogenic Flower Chariot

Not only *Nymphaea* but also *Nelumbo* plants were used in preparing soma. In fact, the *Nelumbo* plant or sacred lotus of India plays an important role in the soma ceremonies of the Ṛg Veda. While the heads of the Aśvins, as well as their horses, are specifically *Nymphaea (puṣkara)* buds or open flowers, the Aśvins' chariot is a combination of both *Nymphaea* and *Nelumbo (puṇdarika)* flowers.

The heads of the twin Aśvins have two important aspects. In some hymns each is said to each be crowned with an opened *Nymphaea* flower. In other hymns each is said to have the head of a horse, represented by a *Nymphaea* flower bud that is unopened, or just about to open. These two characteristics of *Nymphaea* flowers are important not only for the structure of the Aśvins' chariot, but also for the psychoactive potency of their drink.

Nymphaea flowers are unusual in that they frequently produce twin buds on a single stem (Fig. 3). These buds can branch separately from the stem, forming a three-columned plant, or they can extend directly out of a single opened flower.

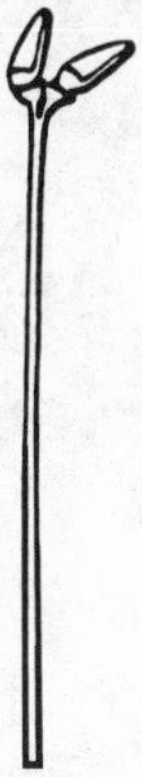

Figure 3.
Dual-budded *Nymphaea* plant as the twin Aśvins.

The chariot of the Aśvins is constructed of the two *Nymphaea* buds, with either a *Nymphaea* flower or a *Nelumbo* flower or flower bud between them. When the *Nymphaea* flower appears between the twin buds, the golden seedpod cut from the *Nelumbo* flower is placed in the center of the opened *Nymphaea* flower by the protégés of the Aśvins. Any one of the combinations of the three flowers used as the chariot forms a triangular shape with a bright golden center. Use of the *Nelumbo* flower, or just its golden seedpod, in the composition of the chariot is due to the *Nelumbo* seedpod's ancient association with the sun in India, an association dating back to the Indus Valley cultures. This becomes apparent when we understand that the Aśvins are responsible for bringing forth the golden dawning sun, as well as other alchemical operations of the sun at the soma ceremony at dawn, noon, and dusk. In addition, the flower chariot is said to be pulled by the Aśvins' horses, which are horse-headed *Nymphaea* plants.

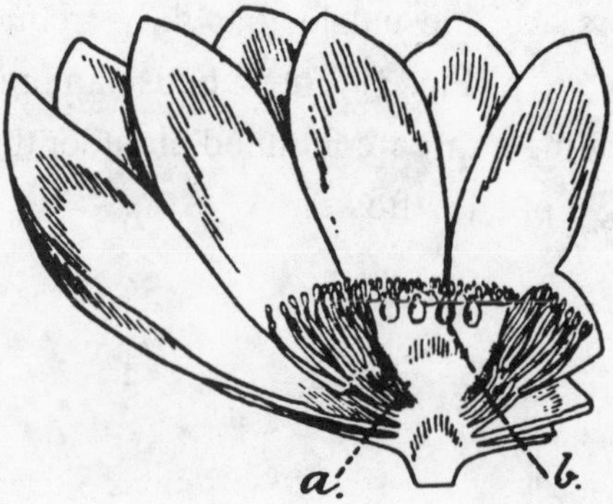

Figure 4. Cross section of *Nelumbo* flower showing (*a*) the triangular-shaped central golden seedpod, and (*b*) the nectar chamber.

In the hymns of the Ṛg Veda, the Aśvins' chariot is said to give the newly born, golden, female sun a ride. This refers to the golden central seedpod of the *Nelumbo* flower (Fig. 4). It was the ancient soma sacrificers known as the three Ṛbhus who originally fashioned the chariot for the Aśvins from the lotus plants. RV 10.39.12 says, "Come forth that chariot which the Ṛbhus made for you Aśvins, that is speedier than thought. At the time of harnessing your chariot [in the morning] heaven's daughter [Uṣas as the sun] springs to birth."

RV 1.194.3 says that the Aśvins' horses come from the waters where Uṣas is born as a bride to join them—the waters being where the day-blooming lotus flowers open in the morning, revealing the newborn golden sun within. The sun rides in the chariot up to the top of heaven at midday and downward to dusk, when the lotus flower closes, shutting off the light of the sun.

The Aśvins' chariot is said to be as swift as thought, indicating the consciousness-expanding effects of the soma drink. The flowers of both *Nelumbo* and *Nymphaea* produce a rich psychoactive nectar and oil. The Aśvins' flower chariot is said to be overflowing with golden oil and nectar, or mead. The hymns also say the chariot is loaded with radiant foam *(ṛjikas)* as fermented nectar or mead. The chariot carries the soma *madhu* drink, which is of a golden color because of the golden center of the *Nelumbo* flower.

The Aśvins, Soma, Lotus Plants, and the Ancient Elixir of Immortality

The pressed-out nectar and sap in both *Nymphaea* and *Nelumbo* flowers and other plant parts from these genera were considered soma in the Ṛg Veda. They were not soma substitutes, but rather an integral part of the various drinks prepared during the soma ceremony. In the Ṛg Vedic version of the soma ceremony there are two significant rituals that make the final soma drink entheogenic as well as an elixir of immortality. First, the juice from the soma stalks containing psychoactive compounds is pressed out. Second, just before dawn, the twin Aśvins, or physicians of the gods, appear. They are masters of herbal knowledge that was partly derived from a very ancient group of soma sacrificers called the Ṛbhus. They prepare a form of mead probably related to other forms of Indo-European mead brews. The Aśvins' inebriating concoction is golden and sweet, and *Nelumbo* and *Nymphaea* flowers and flower parts and nectars have been added to it. In addition, the Aśvins' drink was probably fermented and contained an alcohol content anywhere between 2% and 12%. It is not uncommon for sweet-nectar flowers to contain various microorganisms such as yeast that can rapidly ferment juice within a few hours or less. The Aśvins are said to have created *surā*, a fermented drink made from certain species of *Nymphaea* plants.[17] The association of the Aśvins and fermentation is mentioned in at least five hymns.[18] *Surā* is also connected with *madhu* in the Atharva Veda.[19] The *madhu* or *surā* was kept in skins like the ones the Aśvins carry.[20] The Ṛg Veda describes the golden sun as a wineskin that resembles the Aśvins' golden wineskin.[21] It is noteworthy that out of all the gods of the Vedic pantheon, the Aśvins are privileged to drink soma, *surā*, and *madhu.* These drinks were prepared separately as well as in combination during the soma ceremony and were derived from different preparation procedures and different parts of lotus plants. Fresh soma was prepared from the bitter sap of stems and rhizomes, *surā* from fermented leaves and rhizomes, and soma *madhu* from fermented and nonfermented flower nectar and sap. In many passages, *madhu* means soma juice. In the Śatapatha Brāhmaṇa soma and *surā* are mixed together and are known as the drinks of the sun, as Prajāpati. This is similar to the Ṛg Vedic soma ceremony in which the Aśvins' soma drink is derived from the sun lotus and is a mixture of soma and *surā* derived from the two different types of lotus plants, *Nelumbo* and *Nymphaea.*[22] This concurrence in the Śatapatha Brāhmaṇa continues the relationship established in the Ṛg Veda between the Aśvins, soma, *surā,* and the sun in that soma was sometimes a mixed fermented drink in the hymns. The Aśvins' soma additive makes the bitter, fresh soma juice sweet. The hymns say, "Well seasoned *[tīvro]* is the [soma] mixed with *madhu* [sweet nectars], exhilarating among the Sunahotras," and "soma mixed with *surā* becomes strong."[23] The idea of soma being "well seasoned" indicates that the drink is partly fermented, which helps to explain its epithet *tīvro* (strong).

It is from the Aśvins' soma mixtures that the *somarasa,* or elixir of immortality, was derived. Soma as a *madhu* mead drink is directly mentioned in the Ṛg Veda as being drunk by both the Aśvins and priests.[24] The Aśvins sprinkle the sacrificial juice with their soma mead three times a day, and the resulting drink produces ecstasy, spontaneous healing, rejuvenation, longevity, and immortality.[25]

The Aśvins, who are repeatedly said to be wonderworkers, bring medicines to the priests with their honey-whipped mixtures. Through them and their soma drink miracles take place.[26] The Aśvins enable the priests to cross over to immortality and their special mixtures prolong life and are also associated with various paranormal abilities and direct travel to other worlds.[27]

The soma *madhu* of the Aśvins is also said to bestow mental alertness. It invigorates its drinkers and gives bliss and ecstasy. One hymn says, "When Aśvins worthy of our praise, seated in the Father's house, you bring wisdom and ecstasy."[28] Even the Aśvins are said to be in a state of exalted ecstasy from drinking their own soma *madhu.*[29] The Aśvins are said to create devotional ecstasy in the hearts of the priests, who attain joyous entheogenic ecstasy when drinking the *madhu.*[30]

The Aśvins' chariot is called the Madhuvarna (nectar-bearer). The chariot is the drink itself, comprised of the parts of the flowers and the soma sap nectar from their nectar chambers. Because of this, the chariot alone is said to bring ecstasy. As one hymn says, "For ecstasy I call the ecstatic bestowing chariot, at morning, the inseparable Aśvins with their chariot, I call like Sobhari our father." The chariot, loaded with *madhu,* arrives "rapid as thought, strong and speeding to grant ecstasy."[31] The ecstasy, exaltation, and bliss are all attributes of a divine hallucinogen or entheogen.

The Aśvins have close ties with the Greek Dioscuri, twins who are said to have been aliens to Attica and probably came from India, or are at least of Indo-European descent. The Athenians adopted the twins and then included them into the greater mysteries. They are usually depicted with star-shaped flowers on their heads, just like the Aśvins. On a striking Attic vase of the fifth century B.C.E. that portrays the mysteries, the figures of the Dioscuri can be seen. It is thought that their association with Eleusis may have arisen from some actual part that their statues played in the mystic ritual.[32] Since entheogenic plants were used in the Eleusinian Mysteries, the Dioscuri probably played the same role there as the Aśvins do in the more ancient soma ceremony, that is, as a representation of psychoactive plants that form a special drink that is mixed with other beverages or consumed alone for various healing and entheogenic effects.

The food of the gods is the divine soma mead. It is a special form of soma drink created when soma is mixed with the Aśvins' flower nectar. The gods live and maintain their immortality by drinking this visionary nectar, *amṛta* (ambrosia or mead). "I have partaken wisely of the *[madhu]* sweet food, that stirs good thoughts, best banisher of trouble, the food round which all deities and mortals, calling it nectar-mead, collect together."[33]

In the Ṛg Veda, Tvaṣṭṛ, the artisan of the gods and creator of all forms, is said to drink the special soma mead.[34] His drink is connected to paranormal methods of direct creation. Like the alchemists, the Aśvins are associated with the morning dew. In India, where the dew is heavy, the lotus flowers contain extra amounts of nectar mixed with the dew.[35]

The terms *madhu* and *soma* are both mentioned as the drink to which the Aśvins are invited, and the two are synonymous throughout the Ṛg Veda: "These are soma for you to drink madhu."[36] Soma is specifically said to be a *madhu* drink, and the Aśvins, their color, their chariot, and their horses are all called *madhu.* Thus, the entire *madhu* soma drink comes from the Aśvins.

The Aśvins' soma-mead mixture was prepared at dawn, when different lotus plants are either blooming or closing. This was seen as an alchemical union of the dual principles of day and night, personified as the sun and moon. This union of sun and moon created the drink that induced the experience of light as Anthropos within the priests.

Because of the blooming cycles of the various *Nelumbo* and *Nymphaea* plants used, these genera were once known in ancient India as sun and moon plants. This is one reason why in the earliest Vedic literature, namely, the Ṛg Veda, Atharva Veda, Sāma Veda, and Yajur Veda, soma was associated with both the sun and moon. Beginning with the Brāhmaṇas and early Upaniṣads (900 B.C.E.) soma became increasingly associated with only the moon. The original sun plants of ancient lore were the day-blooming *Nelumbos* and *Nymphaeas.* The moon plants were the night-blooming *Nymphaeas* (there are no night-blooming *Nelumbos*). The Aśvins combined the day- and night-blooming *Nelumbo* and *Nymphaea* together as an alchemical union of the sun and moon plants to produce the elixir of life.

The Aśvins' union of the sun and moon plants in the Ṛg Veda soma ceremony is not only the oldest written form of the creation of the original elixir of immortality, it is also the oldest documented alchemical ritual for producing the "elixir of life." This knowledge is very ancient and is found in the oldest parts of the Ṛg Veda associated with the soma ceremony, as well as in the art of the Indus Valley cultures. It is the probable origin of the union of the sun and moon motif found in European alchemical traditions.

5
SOMA AND THE ORIGINS OF ALCHEMY

Evidence indicates that the Ṛg Vedic soma and soma ceremony lie close to the origins of the world's alchemical traditions. To the best of my knowledge this connection has never been discussed before. In fact, the evidence suggests that the soma tradition may well be the oldest systematic form of alchemy in the world.

India was known from ancient times to be in possession of the elixir of immortality and the fountain of youth. It was even thought to be the site of the earthly paradise and the beginning of the creation of life, as well as the origin of the primordial first man. The origin of the English word man is derived from the Sanskrit name Manu, the first man.

According to the Greek physician Ktesias, who served as personal physician to the Persian king Artaxerxes Mnemon from 405 to 397 B.C.E., the fountain of youth was located in India. Ktesias says of the inhabitants of India, "They are just, and of all men are the longest lived, attaining the age of 170 and some even of 200 years."[1] According to Middle Eastern tradition, Alexander the Great went to India to search for the "water of life."[2] In 326 B.C.E. Nearchus, the admiral of Alexander's fleet in India, described the Indians in his journals as healthy, "free from disease, and living up to a very old age."[3] Onesikritus of Astyplaia was the Greek pilot of Alexander's fleet. He also accompanied Alexander into India and kept a journal of his experiences and observations. He wrote that Indians "live 130 years without becoming old, for if they die then they are cut off as it were in mid-life."[4] Around 321 B.C.E., the Greek ambassador Megasthenes went to India and served for the Seleucid Empire at the court of Chandragupta. Megasthenes wrote a book about India based on firsthand observation in which he mentions the long life span of Indians. He tells us that the Greek myth of the Hyperboreans was of Indian origin. He mentions that these Indian Hyperboreans "live a thousand years." He also says that wine was never drunk by the Indians except at sacrifices when soma juice was consumed. This indicates that at this time soma was a fermented drink.[5] Sedlar speculates that the Greeks did not use the term *soma* to avoid confusion because it meant "body" or "corpse" in Greek.[6] There is also evidence among the Greek historians that the Indians used some form of supernatural means to rejuvenate themselves and to heal the sick. Arrian, a Greek historian and philosopher born toward the end of the first century C.E., compiled from the most reliable sources an account of the Asiatic expedition of Alexander the Great. He noted that when the Greeks felt "themselves much indisposed, they applied to their sophists [Brahmins] who by wonderful, and even more than human means, cured whatever would admit of cure."[7]

As early as the third century B.C.E., Chinese tradition tells of the emperors of China sending expeditions into India and the West in search of the fabled paradise, the plant of immortality, and the elixir of life.[8] There is ample evidence that early Chinese knowledge of the Indian soma motivated the searches of the emperor Ch'in Shih Huang-ti of the Ch'in Dynasty (249–210 B.C.E.) and the emperor Wu-ti of the Han Dynasty (202 B.C.E.–220 C.E.) for the elixir of immortality.[9] Much later, the Chinese pilgrim Pahiyan, while visiting India around 405–411 C.E., was told by the Indian priests that Indians of former ages had long life spans.[10]

Many centuries later the same idea of a miraculous method of increasing longevity found only in India was restated by Marco Polo after his visit to India, circa 1280 C.E. He wrote, "They live to a great age, some of them even to 150 years, enjoying health and vigour . . . although they sleep upon the bare earth."[11]

The location of the original paradise, of the original homeland of mankind, and of the secret of immortality has intrigued humanity for millennia. The original paradise or the Garden of Eden has always been associated with longevity and immortality. Knowledge of the discovery in India of the elixir of immortality and the original Eden of the Bible had reached Europe at least by the twelfth century. Many church fathers and leaders expressed the idea that the original paradise, fountain of youth, and the origin of man were located in India. Some examples are from Saint Athanasius, bishop of Alexandria (300 C.E.), who stated in his *Questionary*, "We are taught that paradise was to the East. . . . For this reason, say the accurate historians, fragrant spices are found in the orient in the direction of India. . . ." Saint Jerome (375 C.E.) pictured paradise as lying somewhere north of India in the Himalayas. In speaking of the original river of paradise that split into four rivers, he writes in his *De sita et nommibus* that "Phison is the river which our Greek scholars call the Ganges. This river pours out of paradise and flows around the regions of India, and finally into the Indian Ocean." In his *De par-*

adiso, Saint Ambrose, archbishop of Milan (400 C.E.), says, "Paradise was planted in the Orient—in a place of delights." He says its source is the Ganges that flows around India.

Legends about India became widely circulated throughout Europe. It was said that not only the fountain of youth but also the much-sought-after origin of creation, the land of Eden, the earthly paradise, was to be found in India. This Indian paradise contained a fountain of youth from which flowed the water of life that could heal the sick and rejuvenate the aged. Europeans were eager to find this place. If the legends were true, then this fountain in paradise would be the key to Adam's longevity and the source of bodily immortality.

In the twelfth century, Hugo of Saint Victor (d. 1142 C.E.) placed the earthly paradise in the East along with its tree of life and fountain of youth:

> Asia has many provinces and regions whose names and locations I shall set forth briefly, beginning with paradise. Paradise is a place in the East, planted with every kind of timber and fruit trees. It contains the tree of life. No cold is there nor excessive heat, but a constantly mild climate. It contains a fountain which runs off in four rivers. It is called paradise in Greek, Eden in Hebrew, both of which words in our language mean a Garden of Delight.[12]

It is interesting that in the Ṛg Vedic soma ceremony four rivers are mentioned. These are the four rivers of paradise that branch off from the single river, which is symbolic of the central pillar/tree of light produced by soma during the ceremony. These rivers of light, equated with a timeless paradise and the fountain of youth, are created by the soma flow at the center of the world where the ceremony is being conducted.

Earlier legends mentioned by Ktesias clearly state that the fountain of youth was located in India. Later, Dion Chrysostom (d. 117 C.E.), in his *Oratio* (25.834), states that the Brahmans of India "possess a remarkable fountain" of youth. Other legends, such as those of Prester John, the mythical Eastern Christian king, also describe paradise as being in India. The paradise of Prester John contained a fountain of youth "which preserves health for three hundred and three years, three months, three weeks, and three days."[13] Not only the Christian but also the Islamic tradition placed paradise in India. According to traditions current among the Muslims, Adam, the first man, called *manu* or *man* in Sanskrit, originally descended from heaven to India and received his first revelation there.[14]

All of these stories, myths, and legends are connected to a variety of traditions that existed in ancient India. The source of these legends lies in the traditions and ancient stories in the Ṛg Veda that discuss rejuvenation. The rejuvenation stories found in the Ṛg Veda are the oldest written sources that we possess concerning the rejuvenation of humans rather than gods, goddesses, or serpents.[15]

The Ṛg Vedic soma ceremony also appears to be the oldest preserved document in which human beings attain immortality while still living in a physical body. The only exception to this is Utnapishtim, who lived with the gods in Dilmun in the garden of the sun and was made immortal after the flood. Another source for the legends derives from eyewitness accounts of travelers exposed to the sages and the long traditions of the saints of India who were renowned for such supernatural abilities as healing the sick, rejuvenating the aged, and personal immortality. The genesis of such stories is the logical outcome of the cosmogony and cosmology developed by the ancient Indians in their earliest literature. This cosmology allowed for the existence of a fundamental constituent of the universe, derived from the source of creation, that could nourish and rejuvenate matter. This special substance was called soma. It maintained the rejuvenating abilities of not only plant and human life, but the earth, sun, moon, planets, and the eternity of the universe as a whole. These early ideas led to the notion that the earthly paradise, the fountain of youth, and the water of life were to be found in India. The origin of these ideas in their fully developed forms are directly connected to the earliest soma ceremonies described in the Ṛg Veda.

Widespread knowledge of soma as an elixir of immortality or "water of life" demonstrates its emergence and diffusion throughout the Ṛg Vedic period and must be at least as old as the oldest hymns, if not older. This would date the soma system of alchemy to around 1800 B.C.E. and make it the oldest developed form of elixir alchemy known. The rituals of the soma ceremony, and soma itself, are used for mystical union and healing in the Ṛg Veda, and they form the foundation of the beliefs in rejuvenation and healing in portions of the Artharva Veda. The soma alchemical system forms the basis of the later alchemical, *rasāyaṇa,* and Ayurvedic schools of India. Parts of this system are also incorporated into the different techniques of yoga and tantra in the Hindu, Jain, and Buddhist schools.

ORIGINS OF THE ELIXIR THEORY OF ALCHEMY

The "water of life" is infrequently mentioned in Sumerian, Babylonian, Assyrian, and Egyptian texts, and it does not appear to have ever been developed in these cultures into either an herbal or specific internal alchemical system as soma was. Nor did mortals ever obtain the immortal status of the gods as they did after drinking soma in the Ṛg Veda. The old Indo-European mead drink reached its fullest development in Indo-Iranian rituals as the ambrosia of the gods. This is specifically true of the Indo-Aryan soma, which became the drink of both the gods and human beings. A number of Ṛg Vedic hymns clearly state that at one time only the gods gained immortality through drinking soma. But through supernormal means, the Atharvans (soma priests) discovered the gods' ancient secret of the preparation of the entheogenic soma drink that allowed human beings to obtain the same immortal status as the gods.

The notion of a substance such as the water of life, later called an alchemical elixir, was systematically formulated among the Indo-Iranians at an early date, possibly as early as 3500 B.C.E. It was the Vedic Aryans, the originators of Sanskrit, the "language of the gods," who called this elixir soma, a Sanskritized form of the Avestan *haoma* drink, and who advanced this elixir idea to a fully developed internal system of alchemy. The priests of the Ṛg Veda considered the celestial elixir that flowed through the trunk of the cosmic tree to be the universal panacea, the water of life that could heal, rejuvenate, and give immortality directly. Interestingly, the theory of an elixir of life did not originally exist in other forms of alchemy that were to develop many centuries later throughout the world. There is strong evidence that the elixir theory in early alchemical traditions was transmitted to these traditions from the early Indo-Iranian sacrificial rituals of soma and *haoma*. The Indian soma, more so than its counterpart *haoma*, was much further developed as the internal elixir and was transmitted to subsequent alchemical traditions. Soma was the original healer, rejuvenator, and life-span extender of ancient civilization. The soma of the Aryans described in the Ṛg Veda is the source of the notion of the elixir of life that influenced the development of the alchemical *elixir vitae* in such diverse cultures as China, Islam, and Europe. The transmutation of base metals into gold may have originated elsewhere; however, there is early and clear evidence that this notion may also have come from the Indo-Iranian sacrificial rituals. This evidence can be clearly seen in the Ṛg Vedic soma ceremony in its teaching of the internal method for inducing paranormal abilities such as psychogenesis (mind-born creations or transmutations). Current research has suggested that elixir alchemy was first developed in China among the Taoists. It can be shown, however, that Chinese elixir theories were derived from the elixir theory in India that came from the Ṛg Veda. The notion of a rejuvenating elixir appears to have been transmitted to China from India at a very early date and from the Chinese and Indians to the Arabs, from which it was transmitted through Arabic alchemical and scientific writings to Jewish philosophers and to Roger Bacon, who disseminated this information throughout Europe around 1250 C.E.[16] Joseph Needham shows that soma was the original alchemical elixir of life in Indian, Chinese, Middle Eastern, and European alchemical texts. Some of these influences came directly from the Ṛg Veda soma ceremony of the Brahmans and the Atharva Veda while others were by way of later Hindu and Buddhist religious and philosophical texts.

My purpose is to show how Indian religion and philosophical doctrines derived from the Ṛg Vedic soma ceremony have influenced Chinese, Greco-Egyptian, and Islamic alchemy, and how they became incorporated into European alchemical texts, practices, and lore.

SOMA AND CHINESE ALCHEMY

Chinese alchemy is primarily concerned with prolonging life and the search for the *elixir vitae*. As noted above, this search for an elixir was carried out by the *ṛṣis* of the Ṛg Veda and other Indian ascetic groups dating back to at least 1800 B.C.E. Some of the practices developed by these sages were completely internal, while others used triggers such as entheogens in conjunction with breathing, sound, and visualization practices. The groups of ascetics known as the *Munis* and the *Kesins*, whose names in Sanskrit mean "silent, long-haired sages," have a special and powerful hymn written about them in the Ṛg Veda. They were great miracle workers who internalized the concepts of the soma sacrifice and perfected the uniting of the opposites of fire and water. By internalizing the soma sacrificial concepts, these ascetics were able to develop a subtle body, identified with the sun as the cosmic pillar/tree, through which they attained immortality. As described in the Ṛg Veda, this solar body was said to exit and return to the physical body, and it was through this solar body that the alchemical elixir soma was drunk. Their deity was the fierce god Rudra, lord of plants. Known as the "red howler," Rudra is directly connected with Indra, Soma, and the sun. The Ṛg Vedic Maruts are Rudra and Indra's companions, and they are associated in both the Ṛg Veda and the Atharva Veda with the seven vital breaths that howl like a whirlwind when leaving the body. The *Munis* and *Kesins* used various herbal concoctions to produce states of ecstasy and were able to leave the body at will.

Another early ascetic group, called the *vrātyas*, were great miracle workers. They internalized the principles of the soma ceremony and practiced special forms of ascesis that are still not completely understood. The *vrātyas*, who were herbal alchemists, also worshipped Rudra, lord of plants. They are said to have searched for and found the elixir of life.[17] Their ascesis involved not just the mortification of the physical body, but a practice based on the internal vibrations *(vipra)* within the matrix (*hṛdyakasa*, or space within the heart), the universal womb of creation associated with the Anthropos. Their practices involved a combination of fasting, breath control, entheogenic drug use, and the internal repetition of phonemes. They entered ecstatic states and cosmicized their subtle bodies into replicas of the universe.

Both Indian ascetics and early texts such as the Ṛg Veda, Atharva Veda, and the Upaniṣads, as well as Buddhism, influenced the development of Chinese alchemy. In both the Ṛg Veda and the Atharva Veda, the elixir was associated with gold, the imperishable solar metal. The emphasis of the Chinese alchemists was placed upon making gold, a substance that would confer longevity or immortality to the body. This idea does not appear to enter Western alchemy until the Islamic period.

Legend has it that Chinese alchemy originated in the teachings of the naturalist school, whose founder was Zou Yan (300 B.C.E.). The naturalist school propagated the yin-yang and five-element theory, but that the idea of an "elixir of immortality" developed from their doctrines without outside influence cannot be shown. As will be discussed later, from before the time of the development of the naturalist school, there was a direct influence upon the development of Chinese alchemy from Indo-Iranian sources with regard to the plant of immortality and the "elixir of life." The oldest treatise in China devoted entirely to alchemy is the *Cantongqi* by Wei Bo-yang, which dates only to about 142 C.E.[18] Taoism, however, can be traced back to its founder, Lao-tzu, who lived around the fourth century B.C.E.[19] Taoist alchemy, much like its Indian counterpart, became associated with all manner of wonder-working and magic. Early on, its attention was focused on the problem of mortality. By bringing the body into a perfect harmony with the Tao, the way of the universe, the body would acquire the attributes of the Tao and so become deathless. The concept of the Tao is not different from the Ṛg Vedic concept of *ṛta*, the foundation of eternal order, the principle of universal harmony and balance at the cosmic center of being. This principle operates throughout all of nature in both its animate and inanimate forms.

There are many similarities between the Ṛg Vedic soma and Chinese alchemy. In both Chinese alchemy and European alchemy, the elixir or philosopher's stone undergoes various color changes to reach perfection. The soma of the Ṛg Veda goes through similar color changes during the soma ceremony, including black, symbolic of primal matter before creation, and then various shades of white, gold, red, and purple or rainbow colors. In the soma ceremony, the color of the soma juice was alchemically altered by the priests from white before dawn to a golden color after dawn until midday (by the union of white and reddish yellow) and then to reddish yellow in the evening. These same color changes in the matter of the philosopher's stone are found in Chinese, Islamic, and European alchemy.

In China the language of alchemy was applied to various techniques of breath control whose aim was also physical immortality. The goal of the practices was the resurrection of the integral personality in a new and imperishable body form, a body of light. In Chinese alchemy this special body was nurtured like an embryo within the physical body by yogic disciplines. The European alchemist, working along the same lines, brings an elixir to maturity in a matrix of lead. The development of a new, embryonic, imperishable body inside the physical body is derived from the soma ceremony of the Ṛg Veda. Within the matrix of the heart-cave-womb in the soma ceremony a golden embryo is generated that becomes the internal body of light or Anthropos.

Special breathing techniques are first encountered in the Ṛg Vedic soma ceremony with the chanting of sacred syllables by the *ṛṣis* and during their practice of generating internal heat and light. The Ṛg Vedic hymns were written in a variety of magical chanting meters. The rhythmic monotony of these incantations was accompanied by breathing techniques specific to each meter; the method of chanting each meter was a well-kept secret. The ritual development of the embryonic alchemical sun within the womb is a special part of the Ṛg Vedic soma ceremony that employed special breathing techniques *(tapas)* associated with fire and sound. In the Atharva Veda there are detailed examples of methods of embryonic womb breathing. The healing power is said to reside in the breath, remaining latent until stimulated according to the established magical ritual.

A number of Chinese alchemists used Indian breathing (Sanskrit *prana*, Chinese *chi*) techniques in their practices. Some of these are Lu Pu-wei (d. 237 B.C.E.), Liu An (d. 122 B.C.E.), and Hua T'o (189 C.E.). Hua T'o was a famous physician and master of life energy *(chi)*. Hua T'o's techniques have been shown to be derived from India. Even his name is derived from a transliteration of a Sanskrit word for medicine, *agadya*, which means "universal cure-all."[20] Breathing techniques themselves are a very ancient tradition in China, certainly older than Chinese alchemy itself.[21] Even though breath or *chi* control practices were being used in China already in the sixth century B.C.E.,[22] the Indian counterpart to such practices dates from the hymns in the Ṛg Veda, Atharva Veda, Brāhmaṇas, Āraṇyakas, and Upaniṣads, which places the use of these techniques in India at least before 1200 B.C.E. And since the generation of the solar embryo with special breathing techniques is present in the early development of the Ṛg Vedic soma ceremony as an integral component, this could push the above date back to 1800 B.C.E. or even earlier. Portions of the Atharva Veda can be dated to before 1150 B.C.E. by the mention of iron in the text. Other parts are much older and incorporate yoga-type practices, breathing techniques, and medicinal knowledge from indigenous Indian cultures.

The great French Indologist Jean Filliozat addressed the question of whether Taoist breath control antedates the corresponding Indian yogas. He suggests that while each system is peculiar to its culture, there are too many similarities to argue entirely independent development. At the same time, he is convinced that such common elements as the concern with retention of the pneuma or breath and the use of certain positions go back too far in India and must have been imported directly into China.[23]

The embryonic respiration described in Taoist texts is more like the early forms found in the Ṛg Vedic soma ceremony and must be derived from the latter. As noted by Mircea Eliade, "The embryonic respiration (of the Chinese) was not, therefore, like *prāṇāyāma*, an exercise preliminary to meditation, nor an auxiliary technique, but sufficed in itself . . . to set in motion and bring to completion a 'mystical physiology' which led to the indefinite prolongation of life of the material body."[24] This is exactly what we find as the goal of the creation of the subtle body in the Ṛg Vedic soma ceremony. Within the creative matrix of the universal womb the golden embryo is nurtured and brought to full development. It does not involve a continued *prāṇāyāma* regimen of breathing exercises, yet internal fiery breath within the womb plays a vital part. These techniques may have been part of the religious practices of the Indus Valley cultures (2700 B.C.E.), where seal impressions have been found that depict sages seated in yogic postures. It is now known that the Indus Valley cultures were in direct contact with central Asia (Bactria), which was the original homeland of the Indo-Iranians. In the Ṛg Veda itself womb breathing is associated with the ecstasy states of the soma ceremony and the heart-sun-womb of one's internal being. The drawing in and breathing out of rays as breaths from the solar heart is a basic component of the practice described there.

As we have shown, there is overwhelming evidence that the Chinese Taoist rejuvenation and longevity techniques have their origin in the Ṛg Veda and Atharva Veda, which far predate any Chinese Taoist or alchemical texts. The soma ceremony described in both the Ṛg Veda and the Atharva Veda is the source of the elixir theory, the practice of embryonic womb breathing, various psychogenic processes, other breathing exercises, and the concept of the breath as an energy source in the universe.

Another important idea derived from the Ṛg Vedic soma ceremony is the association between the Pole Star and Big Dipper and the heavenly elixir and rejuvenation and longevity concepts. The Pole Star and Big Dipper figure in the archaic myths of most cultures, but their use as the source and holder of the elixir of immortality in a developed cosmogony and cosmology comes from the soma ceremony of the Ṛg Veda. In India from an early date, kingship was associated with the Pole Star in an older form of cosmology involving the deity Varuṇa.

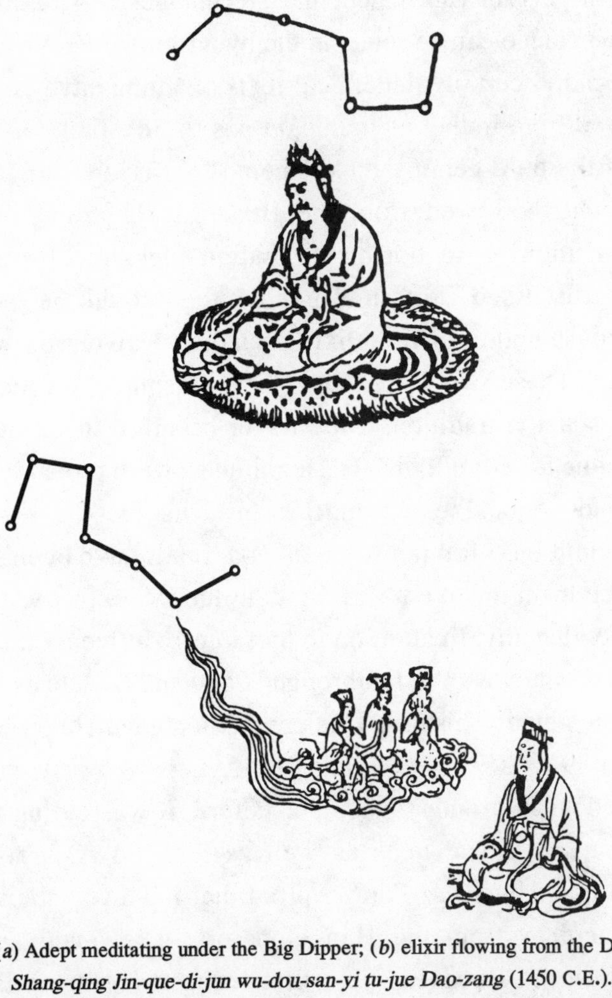

a.

b.

Figure 5. (*a*) Adept meditating under the Big Dipper; (*b*) elixir flowing from the Dipper, from *Shang-qing Jin-que-di-jun wu-dou-san-yi tu-jue Dao-zang* (1450 C.E.).

There is evidence in the Indus Valley culture and in the Ṛg Veda that associates not only Varuṇa but also Indra and Soma with the Pole Star. Indra, the main deity of the hymns who plays an essential role in the soma sacrifice, actually replaces Varuṇa as the Pole Star during the soma ceremony: Varuṇa is said to become Indra.[25]

In China, according to Confucian philosophy, the Pole Star was also associated with kingship. Both the Pole Star and the Big Dipper are prominent aspects of Taoist alchemical techniques, and it is highly likely that their source can be found in the hymns of the Ṛg Veda (Fig. 5).

Furthermore, certain alchemical texts of China have been directly borrowed from Indian alchemical texts. An example of this is the writing of the third-century-C.E. alchemist Ko-Hung, surnamed Pao-p'u tzu, who borrowed from the Buddhist Nāgārjuna's *Rasaratnācara.* In addition to borrowing Indian alchemical knowledge, Ko-Hung discussed certain miracles that could be performed through consumption of the elixir, including walking on water and levitation.[26] These two feats have only one source, the Indo-Aryan Ṛg Veda *somapa* tradition. They never occurred in China prior to their introduction from India. These miracles were probably incorporated into alchemical texts from Buddhist sources.

The ancient Indo-Iranian soma/*haoma* rituals have been shown by Joseph Needham to have had a direct influence on the development of Chinese alchemy. In addition to these early influences, there was continuous contact with India through Hindu and Buddhist envoys, as recorded in Chinese history. This contact included Hindu envoys of 105 B.C.E., 89 B.C.E., 159 C.E., and 161 C.E., as well as the introduction of Buddhism around 2 B.C.E. or before. It was during this span that Indian alchemical texts as well as texts on respiration were translated into Chinese.[27] Further proof that India was the source of the elixir comes from the Han emperors, who, upon asking for instruction in the Buddhist faith, first requested that the Buddhists supply them with the "herbal elixir of immortality," which only India was known to possess.[28] In India, however, the elixir ideas associated with immortality were more greatly developed than in the Iranian Avesta. As mentioned by Lu Gwei-Djen, India appears to have been the original influence upon Chinese alchemy's development of physiological alchemy or *nei tan*, which is a quasi-yogistic system of internal alchemy in which an elixir of immortality is synthesized within the body of the alchemist.[29] The ancient soma plant of the Ṛg Veda also had an influence on the development of Chinese herbal alchemy. Chinese sages are known to have sought a special plant in India—which had to be soma—that was supposed to bestow healing, longevity, and immortality. Not only did the Chinese emperors of the Ch'in and Han Dynasties seek out the soma plant of India, but one of the oldest Chinese medical texts, *Pen-ts'ao Kang Mu*, mentions a lotus plant called *hung-pai-lien-hua*, which was from a foreign country and considered the plant of immortality. We can attribute the many parallels between Chinese alchemy and the elixir theories of immortality found in early Indian texts directly to the influence of Indian elixir theories on Chinese philosophy.

The Ṛg Vedic soma ceremony includes within itself cosmic processes and cycles of creation, maintenance, and destruction that are models for alchemical processes. The soma of the soma ceremony is a combination of entheogenic plant juices and pneumatic development within the body of the adept. The process of developing an etherealized subtle body within the heart is the foundation of the soma ceremony. This imperishable body, which is able to remain in the physical body or to leave it behind, is used for healing, longevity, paranormal abilities, and immortality. The Atharva Veda is full of hymns that tell of the leaving of the physical body through an internal, golden, subtle form generated within the womb of the heart. This concept, and the meaning of the soma ceremony as an early form of internal alchemy, has not been fully appreciated or understood by scholars of the origins of alchemy.

The ritual processes of the soma ceremony not only developed a special internal body in the adept but also gave the adept the capacity for psychogenesis and other psychic abilities. We find in the soma ceremony that the soma elixir not only creates an immortal subtle body of light but also is the method by which miracles are conducted. In the soma ceremony there is a process in which the mind and the heart are combined during the ritual in order to access the matrix continuum called the *skambha*. The matrix continuum is the creative, universal womb located within the heart of being. This continuum-womb is identical to the Islamic philosopher's egg, the internal elixir embryo of Taoist alchemy, and the Hermetic vessel of European alchemy. These ideas originally come from the Ṛg Vedic soma ceremony.[30] For example, Joseph Needham says that "the alchemist undertook to contemplate the cycles of cosmic process in his newly accessible form because he believed that to encompass the Tao with his mind (or, as he would have put it, his mind-and-heart) would make him one with it. That belief was precisely what made him a Taoist."[31] This combining of heart and mind is also central to the soma ceremony. "Looking at all the evidence impartially, one cannot escape the conclusion that the dominant goal of proto-scientific alchemy was contemplative, and indeed the language in which the elixir is described was ecstatic."[32] This also shows a close correlation to the ecstatic states attained by the priests that are mentioned in the Ṛg Vedic soma ceremonies.

The motivation of both the first emperor of the Ch'in Dynasty, Ch'in Shih Huang-ti, and Wu-ti of the Han Dynasty for seeking the elixir of immortality comes from Indo-Iranian sources,[33] and, more specifically, from the Ṛg Veda and the Atharva Veda, where the ideas were formulated into a coherent system of internal alchemical practice, a fact that is not the case for the Iranian Avesta.

The soma practices of India were all that was needed to trigger the development of elixir alchemy in Taoist China. Joseph Needham has mentioned that China in the Warring States, Chin, and Han periods would have provided precisely the supersaturated solution from which elixir alchemy would crystalize, given the right seed. Fifty years ago H. H. Dubs proposed that this seed was knowledge of (or hearsay about) the Indo-Iranian plant used by priests in their sacrifices late in the second millennium B.C.E. Called *haoma* by the Persians and soma by the Indians, its use must antedate the Aryan invasions because it is firmly attested to by both Avestan and Vedic sources. The juice of this plant was believed, as far as one can tell from the phraseology of the hymns, to cure all diseases of body and mind and to confer immortality. Dubs went on to suggest that the means of transmission to China was through the Yueh-Chih people, who occupied western Kansu down to the third century B.C.E., and whose chief city was Kanchow (modern Changyeh). This is the people, in fact, whose alliance Chang Chien went to seek in Han Wu-ti's time after they had moved further to the west. Thus Dubs envisaged an overland transmission of the idea of the drug or plant of immortality from the Indo-Iranian cultural area to China early in the fourth century B.C.E., if not before.[34] Evidently we have here something far more concrete than the metaphors of the Greco-Egyptian protochemists, and something that would have supplied just the element necessary to make the Chinese Taoist set of ideas gel into full elixir alchemy.[35] How this could have come about, according to Needham, can be seen most strikingly if we examine ancient Indian liturgical texts, where the essential germ of alchemy is defined as the art of long life plus aurifaction, noting, by the way, that the connection of the idea of eternal life with the incorruptible metal gold was probably a good deal older. It is easy to say that this connection must go back to the very first knowledge of the properties of metals. When one looks for it in texts from ancient Egypt or

Mesopotamia, there is not much to be found.[36] What is much more important is the remarkable fact that in ancient India gold was intimately bound up with the soma sacrifice itself.[37] Such then, it would seem, is the background both of the "plant of immortality" that Ch'in Shih Huang-ti sought and the alchemical gold that Li Shao-Chun undertook to manufacture. Surely some rumor or persuasion of a most compelling character, reaching China from Indo-Aryan sources, turned divinity into philosophy, or, to speak more precisely, liturgiology into protoscience.[38]

The Chinese continued to consider India as the main source for the knowledge of the "elixir of life" and sent many missions there in order to bring back specific persons who could prepare the elixir for the emperor. In 648 C.E., the emperor T'ai Tsung sent to India the envoy Wang Hsüan-tsē, who brought back a Brahman named Narayanaswamy who was a specialist in "prolonging life." In 664–65 C.E. the Buddhist monk Hsüan-chao was ordered by Kao Tsung to bring from Kashmir one Lokāditya, who possessed the herbal drug of longevity. Lokāditya remained at the Chinese court at least until 668 C.E.[39]

India continued to influence Chinese alchemical ideas through the introduction of Buddhism.[40] After the development of Chinese alchemy, the elixir ideas of soma and the soma ceremony continued to influence other cultures, particularly Islam. The ideas of soma were passed on to Islam indirectly through Chinese alchemy and directly by contact with India.

Soma and Greco-Egyptian Alchemy

There are traditions that claim the origin of alchemy was in Egypt. But like the Gnostic schools and the Hermetic literature, alchemy as formulated in Egypt was a syncretic philosophical system developed from many sources. The foundation of much of the spiritual dimension of Greco-Egyptian alchemy comes from Indo-Iranian sources.

An important figure in Greco-Egyptian alchemy was Demokritos (460–370 B.C.E.), who is said to have traveled widely and is thought to have spent time in India.[41] Demokritos is recalled mainly as the founder, with Leukippos, of the atomic theory, according to which all bodies are made of atoms that are themselves complete, indivisible, simple, eternally existent in empty space, but differing in form and magnitude, with proportional weight. All change comes through combinations or dissociations of atoms in a purely mechanical way. The atomic theory is closely associated with alchemy in its creation and transmutation aspects. The atomic theory was already known in India by the Ājīvikas, an ascetic sect of miracle workers that existed before and at the time of the Buddha, around 500 B.C.E. From what we know of his life, Demokritos appears to have lived as an ascetic. It is very possible that he obtained his atomic theory from India. He also believed in a void, a purely Ṛg Vedic concept found in the soma ceremony and later taken over by the Buddhists. In addition, he said that souls were soul-atoms and that the soul consisted of smooth spherical storms of fire, a concept directly related to the fiery pneumatic body in the heart where the soul resides. These same ideas are found among the theological concepts of the Ājīvikas and are derived from the soma ceremony.

Demokritos was interested in much more than atoms. An entire alchemical school formed around him and his ideas. The Greek author Pliny consistently links Demokritos with the Magi of Persia. Pliny notes that Demokritos wrote an important book about plants in which he says that he will start with the magical wonder plants. According to Pliny, these magical plants were first brought to the notice of the West by Pythagoras and Demokritos, who invoked the

Magi as their authority. The magical plants mentioned by Demokritos mainly are connected with altered states of consciousness and are derived from the *haoma* and soma plants of Persia and India.[42]

During the formulation of alchemy in Greco-Roman Egypt in the first and second centuries C.E., there were direct trade links with India. A statuette found at Pompeii of the Hindu goddess Lakṣmī, who is associated with the lotus plant, has been dated to this time.[43] According to Greek sources, the Persian mystic and magus Ostanes (500 B.C.E.) was the first to explain both magic and alchemy to the Greco-Egyptians. According to Pliny, he was the first writer on magic and a direct pupil of Zoroaster. Ostanes was obviously an Indo-Iranian well acquainted with the magical/alchemical rituals of the entheogenic *haoma*/soma ceremonies.

Very important Greco-Egyptian magicians and alchemists were said to be Ostanes' disciples. These included "Maria the Jewess," who wrote several important books on alchemy, as well as the famous Demokritos himself.[44] One other very influential writer associated with Greco-Egyptian alchemy is Poisidonius (135–51 B.C.E.) from Apamea in Syria. He was head of the Stoic school at Athens and was responsible for many Stoic doctrines. He blended science with astrology, magic, and alchemy. He was directly influenced by Indo-Iranian thought and fused Greek philosophy with Indo-Iranian sacrificial mysticism.[45]

We find ideas identical to those of the Ṛg Vedic soma ceremony in books ascribed to Ostanes. He describes seven gates through which the goal of gnosis can be reached; he goes on to say that the land of Egypt is superior to all others on account of its wisdom and knowledge. The people of Egypt as well as those of the rest of the world, however, have need of the inhabitants of Persia and cannot succeed in any of their works without the aid that they draw from this country. All the philosophers who have devoted themselves to the science of alchemy have addressed themselves to persons from Persia whom they have adopted as brothers.[46]

The main ideas that were transmitted through Greece and Egypt concern the Indo-Iranian sacrificial rituals of *haoma*/soma. These rituals involve an up-and-down motion and circulation process, both within the human body and the greater universe. The notion of up-and-down movement is important in Greek alchemy. It has a direct relationship to uniting the aspects of microcosm and macrocosm. Another important part of the sacrificial rituals is the concept of the spiritual water. The subtle water is the luminous soma energy or fiery water. This water is both the source of the unification of opposites and the ultimate goal of the alchemical quest. The sacrificial ritual unites the above and the below and opens up the source of the light of lights. All of these Greco-Egyptian alchemical operations take place within the bowl-shaped altar as the alembic-womb of transformation. This universal matrix is located at the cosmic center within the heart of being. An understanding of the Greek alchemist Zosimos can be achieved only by an understanding of the Indo-Iranian sacrificial rituals, especially the soma ceremony. During the soma ceremony a dismemberment and then a rememberment occur within the solar heart, the Hermetic vessel. Within the heart as the alembic-womb, luminous rays of being are gathered together through the sensory channels and alchemical creations and transmutations are formed within the oceanic-pneumatic matrix and projected from the heart outward into manifestation.[47]

Soma and Islamic Alchemy

The Islamic world was affected by China, Greece, and India. Both China and Greece had incorporated ideas about soma, and through direct contact with India, the elixir theory entered Islamic thought, having a measurable impact upon Islamic alchemy. Impressed with Indian learning, the Arabs incorporated many Indian ideas into Islamic alchemical texts. Relations between India and the Arabs go back far before the rise of Islam. From among all the cultures with which the Arabs came into contact, they were most impressed by the Greeks and the Indians. According to 'Amr b. Bahr al-Jahiz of Basra (d. 869 C.E.), "I have found the inhabitants of India to have made great advancement in astrology and mathematics. In the science of medicine also they are highly advanced. The Chinese do not possess the qualities which they have. . . . With them originated mysticism and charms which counteract poisons. The origin of astronomical sciences goes back to the Indians."[48]

Another important Arabic author, the well-known historian al-Ya Qubi (d. 900 C.E.), remarks, "The Indians are men of science and thought. They surpass all other peoples in every science; their judgement on astronomical problems is the best; and their book on this subject is the *Siddhanta* which has been utilized by the Greeks as well as the Persians and others. In the science of medicine their ideas are highly advanced. . . ."[49]

Still another great Arabic writer of the ninth century, Abu Ma-shar al-Balkhi (d. 885 C.E.), says, "The Indians are the first (most advanced nation). All the ancient peoples have acknowledged their wisdom and accepted their excellence in the various branches of knowledge. The kings of China used to call the Indian kings, 'the kings of wisdom,' because of their great interest in the sciences."[50]

Many Indian physicians came to Arabia and not only practiced medicine but helped in the translation of Indian medical and philosophical texts from Sanskrit to Arabic.[51] As one Tamil work states, "One of the Siddhars of Tamilnadu, Ramadevar, says in his work on alchemy that he went to Mecca, assumed the name of Yakub and taught the Arabians the alchemical art. It is significant that some of the purification processes and substances of alchemical significance are common to both the Islamic and the Indian alchemy."[52]

Living in the later part of the eighth century, Geber (Jābir), an Arab alchemist and Sufi, is credited with the formulation of the famous sulphur/mercury theory of alchemy. The sulphur/mercury theory is probably of foreign origin, because it occurs in the oldest Chinese alchemical text, *Cantongqi*, written in 142 C.E. by Wei Bo-yang.[53] In India the theory can be traced back to the Ṛg Vedic soma ceremony, where the Aśvins produce a golden elixir composed of sun and moon lotus plants by the union of Agni (fire) and Soma (water). Many eighth-century alchemical manuscripts written in Arabic, Syrian, and Persian abound in references to the sulphur/mercury theory. Through their eventual translation into Latin by European scholars around the beginning of the twelfth century C.E., much of the academic knowledge of the Arabs, including the sulphur/mercury theory, was transmitted to Western Europe. The sulphur/mercury theory of alchemy was really an attempt to show in chemical terms the union of opposite natures in the production of the Grand Elixir. In sixteenth-century Europe, the sulphur/mercury theory was expanded to include salt, which then became known as the triune microcosm. These three principles form the backbone of much of European alchemical speculation.

"According to Latin as well as Arabic books, Geber was surnamed El-Sufi, the Sufi. He acknowledges in his works the Imam Jafar Sadiq (700–765 C.E.) [the great Sufi teacher] as his master." Geber "was for a long time a close companion of the Barmecides, the viziers of Haroun el-Rashid. These *barmakis* [as they were called] were descended from the priests of the Afghan Buddhist shrines, and were held to have at their disposal the ancient teaching that had been transmitted to them from that area."[54] Geber's philosophical views were no doubt greatly influenced by his contacts with the

Barmecides, who were also the priests of the fire temple of Balkh, located in Harran, and associated with the Sabians. This reveals another source of Indian alchemical ideas transmitted to the West through the teachings of the Sabians of Harran, who had close relations with India. According to Al-Maśūd, the ancient Sabians went on pilgrimage in the land of Sindan to a temple of Saturn, built by the Indian Māshān, in the city of Al-Mansūrah. This city was situated in ancient times along the old channel of the Indus and was called Brahmanabad by the Indians. It was about one hundred miles south of the Indus Valley city of Mohenjo Daro.[55]

The knowledge the Barmecides transmitted was the ancient wisdom of the Hindus and Buddhists. This information had come by way of the various trade routes connecting Afghanistan to central Asia and India. Shamanism, Hinduism, and Buddhism contributed to the formation of the wisdom of the area.

The entire sulphur/mercury theory of alchemy has its probable antecedents in the Indian philosophy of the Ṛg Veda. It was in the alchemy of the soma ceremony that a structure was developed that created a separation in the original unity of light, which was then restored by the ritual of the soma ceremony. The symbolic union of fire and water, as Agni/Soma, occurs within the heart of the priest during the ceremony in a special alchemical process that culminates in a transmutation of being, granting immortality on the one hand, and the actual abilities of psychogenic creation and transmutation on the other.

The separation and union of the duality of Agni/Soma in the Ṛg Veda is the origin of all Indian speculation on the union of opposites. It is also the probable origin of the dualism found in Islamic alchemical texts. This knowledge from India was probably transmitted to Islamic thought from Greece and China, both of which had already been influenced by Indian philosophy. As noted by H. E. Stapleton, "The dualistic Yin/Yang theory found in Chinese alchemy and philosophy has been shown to be another influence upon China from Indo-Iranian sources. Dualist theories are much older in Indo-Iranian religion than in China."[56] This makes it likely that Indo-Aryan dualist theories of Agni/Soma are the original precursor of the sulphur/mercury theory. It was also transmitted by direct influence from India itself. Paracelsus later added salt to the sulphur/mercury duality for chemical reasons; salt was also a substance that represented the body as the medium in which the two contraries could unite.

European writers have looked on Geber as the founder of the alchemical art, but recent research seems to show that alchemical books attributed to him are another case of attributing the work of many hands to a single legendary figure. Under Geber's name appear numerous treatises; most of them are alchemical, but others cover medicine, astronomy, astrology, magic, mathematics, music, and philosophy. All together they indeed constitute an encyclopedia of the sciences. Still, it has recently been maintained that no Arab author mentions Geber until two centuries after the time in which he was supposed to have lived. It is now regarded as very probable that this vast body of writings was composed by the members of a group that resembles in its religious leanings the secret sect of nature philosophers who called themselves Ikwan al-Safa, a name that has been variously translated as the "Brethren of Purity" or the "Faithful Friends." The Brethren of Purity composed an encyclopedic collection of letters much resembling the Geberian writings. We may suppose then that a sect with a strong belief in the power of science to purify the soul ascribed the works of its members to the legendary Geber.[57] In other words, the Geberian writings, although not without a chemical basis, are really concerned with spiritual alchemy and personal transmutation. This follows closely the origin of alchemical ideas and their deep spiritual nature. As the soma ceremony reveals, the alchemical processes are internal and spiritual.

Indian sciences, therefore, came to play an important part in the growth of the sciences in Islam, a part far greater than is usually recognized. In zoology, anthropology, mathematics, astronomy, and in certain aspects of alchemy, the tradition of Indian and Persian sciences was dominant, as can be seen in the *Epistles (Rasa'il)* of the Brethren of Purity and the translations of Ibn Muqaffa'. It must be remembered that the words *magic* and *magi* are related, and that according to the legend, the Jews learned alchemy and the science of numbers from the Magi while in captivity in Babylon.[58] It should also be noted, however, that Ammianus Marcellinus, the great Roman historian of the fourth century, tells us that the Magi or Persian priests derived their secret arts from the Brahmans of India.[59] Parts of the Indo-Aryan Ṛg Veda are much older than any Iranian religious text. In fact, several prominent scholars, including Thomas Burrows, have argued that an Indo-Aryan empire existed from northern Syria to the Indus Valley in ancient times. The Iranian branch of the Indo-Europeans moved into the Indo-Aryan territory at a later date as an intrusive element. Therefore, the Indo-Aryan soma ceremony may be older than the Iranian *haoma* ceremony from which it is claimed to be derived. This is especially true if it contains components derived from indigenous India and the Indus Valley cultures.

Islamic alchemy had both a chemical and spiritual side, but it is the spiritual side that really seems to hold out the possibility of transmutation. This idea was clear to many Islamic philosophers as well. The spiritual side of alchemy, rather than just the physical practice, was first revealed by Geber's contemporaries, such as Al-Biruni and Ibn Sina (Avicenna). Both are greatly respected in European alchemical circles. These two adepts accepted the cosmological principles of alchemy while rejecting the possibility of transmutation because of the lack of evidence.[60] The cosmological ideas that make up the spiritual aspects of alchemy are sound. This fact is a clue to the possible spiritual foundations of transmutation, which probably antedate the chemical practices, and the idea is further strengthened by the numerous examples of yogis in India and Sufis in Islam being able to transmute any substance into gold without any chemicals, but through the force of the heart of being. The spiritual-elixir ideas contained within Islamic alchemical texts were to have an important impact upon European alchemy. In addition, Indian ideas were to influence the cosmological structure of the Judaic Kabbalah. These cosmogonic and cosmologic ideas then entered European alchemical texts and made a significant impact upon Western alchemy.

Before discussing the purpose of soma in European alchemy, however, it is important to backtrack a bit and see how soma influenced the development of magic in the West.

6 SOMA AND THE ORIGINS OF WESTERN MAGIC

Although magical incantations are known from primitive, Mesopotamian, Egyptian, and Greek religions, it seems that the Indo-Iranian religions are the source of many ritualized and systematic magical practices in antiquity. It can be documented through textual evidence and artifacts such as seal impressions that Indo-European, and specifically Indo-Iranian, sacrificial rituals are the antecedents of many Near Eastern, Egyptian, and Greek forms of magic.

The origins of systematized magic and magical techniques can be traced back to the Indo-Iranian *haoma*/soma ceremonies. The words *magic*, *magician*, *magus*, and *magi* are all related terms that refer directly to the priests and the magical performances of the Indo-Iranian *haoma*/soma sacrificial rituals. There seems to have been some confusion regarding to whom the terms "Persians" and "magi" referred in antiquity. In many cases, they meant the Indo-Aryans and not the Iranians. Even though the word *magi* was used to refer to both Iranian and Indo-Aryan priests, it is most likely the Indo-Aryans who had the more significant influence upon Greece. According to J. V. Prasek, the title "Aryan" is more properly applied to the peoples called Medes and Persians in ancient literature and inscriptions rather than to the Iranians.[1] In addition, the Medes have been directly connected linguistically with the earlier Indo-Aryan empire of the Mitanni (1500 B.C.E. or earlier).[2] A Babylonian synonym for Medes is Umman Manda. One leader of the Umman Manda mentioned in Hittite texts is Za-a-lu-ti, which is an Aryan name. William Albright has suggested that Za-a-lu-ti was the same man as the "Salitis" who founded the Hyksos Fifteenth Dynasty in Egypt (1800 B.C.E.).[3] This would imply that it was the Indo-Aryans who influenced the Greeks rather than the Iranians. This influence would have been over a long period of time beginning at a very early date. Other Indo-Aryan contacts were to be established later with the Ionian Greeks during the Achaemenian reign of Darius (521–486) B.C.E., when he engaged both Ionian and Indian troops in his army. Cultural exchange could easily have taken place between these two elements.[4]

The magi were to have a significant impact upon Greek culture, especially in magical practices and the use of psychoactive herbs. Herodotus (485 B.C.E.) mentions that the magi or Persian priests are responsible for the royal sacrifices. Xenophon (426 B.C.E.) describes these priests as experts in everything concerning the gods.[5] Heraclitus (550 B.C.E.) in fragment 115 couples together magi (magoi) priests with the Dionysian Bacchoi and priestesses who drink an ecstasy-inducing wine drink, which was probably entheogenic. This coupling together indicates a knowledge by Heraclitus of the *haoma*/soma drink's association with the magi. It is also significant to mention that both Charles Kahn and M. L. West show that Heraclitus was indebted to India rather than to the Iranians for many of his ideas. This points to an influence probably associated with the soma drink and ritual rather than to the *haoma*.[6]

Fritz Graf states that the connection between magical practices and the use of herbal plants, including entheogens, appears in Greek literature in the form of new Greek terminologies such as *pharmakon* (herbal drugs) during the spread of Indo-Iranian beliefs within the Greek world.[7] This indicates that the use of the soma drink in conjunction with the soma ritual was the probable origin of ancient Greek herbal ceremonies used to conduct specific entheogenically induced magical rites. This influence upon Greece was to have important later influences upon magical practices found in Greco-Egyptian, Greco-Roman, and European magic.

The Ṛg Vedic soma ceremony teaches the original methods of these forgotten ancient magical rites much more than its Avestan counterpart does. The internal magical use of these rituals was kept secret, and the meaning and cosmological significance of the ceremonies, especially the soma ceremony of the Ṛg Veda, has not been clearly understood until now.

It is in the classical world that the West first gains an understanding of ancient Indo-Iranian magic and the ritual use of the secret "plant of immortality." In a fragment of a poem by Alcman (650 B.C.E.), a Greek living in Sparta, mention is made of the preparation of a drink from a sacred plant. This plant and its preparation resemble the descriptions given in the Ṛg Veda regarding soma.

In Alcman's fragment 34, the following parallels are mentioned: The author refers to the preparation of a plant's juice taking place on the earth's highest point, just like in the soma ceremony. The juice is of a brilliant color and is prepared in golden vessels, just like soma. The juice of the plant is prepared by women, just as soma sometimes is said to be prepared in the Ṛg Veda. Alcman's plant is connected with the moon. It is associated with fire as well as the pouring out of waters and the cosmic tree. Fire, the moon, and the cosmic tree connect Alcman's plant to soma and the soma ceremony. In addition, there are words in his poem that refer to mixing or stirring. Alcman says that the plant juice is stirred in with milk curds, as is soma juice. There is also the indication that this drink was prepared as a sacrificial offering. The plant is called "imperishable" and is equated to *amṛta*, just like soma. Alcman's plant is called "serpent-slayer," a term associated directly with soma when soma is called Vrtrahan, "slayer of Vṛtra." In the Ṛg Veda, Indra drinks large amounts of soma, which gives him the power to slay the serpent, Vṛtra. Alcman's plant is also connected to the ram, which with the goat is associated with the soma plant. All these parallels suggest that there is some probable connection with the Indo-Aryan soma plant and sacrifice, which had an influence in Sparta and on Alcman's poem.

M. L. West has also mentioned an oriental influence on Alcman's cosmology.[8] Alcman's plant is associated with ambrosia and the moon, and West has shown that the Greek conception of ambrosia and the moon is of Indo-Aryan origin. Although soma is sometimes associated with the moon in the Ṛg Veda, it is mainly in other Indian literature, beginning with the Atharva Veda (1150 B.C.E. and older), that soma is said to fill the moon with ambrosia. These concurrences can also be found in the Brāhmaṇas and early Upaniṣads (900 B.C.E.). West believes that Greek thought had been directly influenced by Indian ideas of soma and the moon, as this conception occurs nowhere else but in Indian literature. Another point of contact between Indian and Greek sources was the philosopher Pherekydes of Syros (600 B.C.E.), the reputed teacher of Pythagoras. According to West, "Pherekydes said the moon produces ambrosia daily, and that the gods feed on it there. In certain of the Vedic hymns, but more commonly and more clearly in the *Brahmanas, Upaniṣads,* and the *Puranas*, we find the idea that the moon is the vessel from which the gods drink *Soma*, the divine liquid that gives immortality. . . . As a drink of immortality, *Soma* is called *amṛta*, which is the equivalent of ambrosia, etymologically as well as in sense."[9]

It has already been mentioned that soma was associated with the moon plants used by the Aśvins, and that the moon's association with soma is due at least in part to the Aśvins using *Nymphaea* moon plants in the preparation of their "elixir of immortality."

Recent investigations by Peter Kingsley have shown that the pre-Socratic philosopher Empedocles, who lived in the fifth century B.C.E., played a crucial role in the development of Western culture. Empedocles' philosophy affected both Greco-Egyptian magic and alchemy.[10] Empedocles acted more like an Indian sage than a Greek. He is said to have performed a number of miracles in front of numerous witnesses, including control over the elements and forces of nature and the resurrection of a young woman who had lain for thirty days without breath or pulse beat.[11] He was also said to have been adept in herbal knowledge, which would have included the use of entheogens derived from Indo-Iranian influences.[12] A direct line of influence and transmission to southern Egypt has been shown to have come from Empedocles and the early Pythagoreans, who were greatly influenced by Indo-Iranian magic derived from the *haoma*/soma ceremonies.

Empedocles spoke of a plant that defended against old age. He was probably referring to an actual plant used by the Indo-Iranian magi in their rejuvenation and immortality rituals. He was probably also referring to an internal experience associated with the ritual use of this plant, which is employed in pneumatic magical practices that include rejuvenation. The Indo-Iranian influence upon Empedocles may be in reference to both a physical and a nonphysical plant. The Indo-Aryans had developed magical rejuvenation rituals using entheogenic drinks that triggered ecstatic internal states. The final rejuvenation effect depended on both the pharmacological agents in the herbal drink and the expression of an internal pneumatic body that acted as an intermediary between physical matter and its non-physical origins. This pneumatic or subtle body was also considered by the Indo-Aryans to be an internal plant. Thus the plant used against aging that Empedocles refers to may be the luminous, internal subtle-body plant entheogenically created during the soma ceremony. It is the Indo-Iranian white *hom,* called the glowing white soma plant in the Ṛg Veda. The ritual for the creation of the internal soma plant is not found in the Iranian material, at least not in any developed form, but is merely referred to along with some of its attributes. It is only in the Ṛg Veda that it was fully developed into a co-functioning external/internal ritual.

The actual plant that Empedocles refers to is probably the entheogenic soma plant that is used to create the internal soma plant of light. Empedocles learned his philosophy and magical practices directly from the magi, and he was considered their disciple even in his own lifetime. It is also thought he was influenced by Indian Buddhism.[13] Another point of direct contact between Empedocles and the Indo-Aryans is reflected in his practice of breath control. The Indo-Aryans developed the specific breathing exercises meant to accompany the internalized rituals at a very early date within the Ṛg Veda and the Atharva Veda. Empedocles could not have learned his pneumatic breathing practices from the Iranians, who did not develop these types of breathing exercises in their rituals. Empedocles must have come into contact with yoga-type teachings, as he is known to have practiced various forms of breath control to accompany his magical practices. According to Diogenes Laertius, "Empedocles experimented in the investigation of respiration, and could hold his breath for a long time. He is reputed to have held himself breathless and to have stopped the beat of his heart for an indefinite time."[14]

As we have shown, breath control and breathing exercises in relation to spiritual practices go back to the soma ceremony and the ascetics of the Ṛg Veda, and to the *vrātyas* of the Atharva Veda, which can be dated at least to 1800 B.C.E. and 1500 B.C.E., respectively. An entire philosophy of breath and winds and their micro- and macrocosmic correlations, fully developed in a cosmological spiritual system, can already be seen in the soma ceremony of the Ṛg Veda. Jean Filliozat has shown very clearly the antiquity of breathing exercises in India, and that they are older than in China, Greece, or anywhere else. Further information on Indian magical practices comes from Apollonius of Tyana, who never ceases to extol the virtues and magical power of the Brahmans of India.[15]

The ritual basis of Indo-Aryan magic as practiced in the Ṛg Vedic soma ceremony was based upon both a solar and a stellar cosmology. It was associated with the breath *(prāṇa)* and the formation of a subtle pneumatic body used for cosmic magical operations, paranormal abilities, rejuvenation, and immortal ascension out of the physical body. The entheogenic soma drink's inner formation of this body, coupled with the soma ritual, not only influenced all Indian religions, but also appears to be the original source of influence upon later Western conceptions of the subtle body.

Soma, Neoplatonism, and Theurgy

In the period from 500 B.C.E. to 200 C.E., Egypt was a melting pot of ideas from various cultures and areas, including India. The Egyptians and Indo-Aryans had close ties, at least as early as the beginning and middle of the second millennium B.C.E. with the Hyksos Aryan invasion and marriage contracts with the Mitanni (1400 B.C.E.). There is also an Indian colony that was known to have existed in the Egyptian city of Memphis around 500 B.C.E.[16] Excavations have uncovered unmistakably Indian votive figurines in the temple of Ptah at Memphis.[17] The rise of the Persian Empire around 500 B.C.E. included both Egypt and western India within its boundaries. There is no doubt that Indian influences could be found in Egypt during the development of the Gnostic schools, the Hermetic texts, Neoplatonism, and Greco-Egyptian alchemy, which took place between 200 B.C.E. and 485 C.E.[18]

The original Ṛg Vedic cosmology that posits the unmanifest world of light and the manifest world of matter as mirror images of each other is very close to both kabbalistic and Neoplatonic metaphysics.[19] These notions were apparently derived from Indian sources.[20] It is this cosmology that gives rise to the conception of the physical creation being an inversion of ultimate reality or the realm of light. This does not really mean that heaven is upside down, as many philosophers in antiquity thought, but rather that the return to the source is a reversal of the normal activity of the senses. One must go inward and not outward to find ultimate reality. Once the connection is established, however, one can still function in the world.

The fundamental example in the Ṛg Veda is the descent from the One during creation as a downward and inverted process, just as a child is born headfirst from its mother. In the cosmogonic act described in the soma ceremony the supernal light of soma that forms matter descends and disperses during the creation process. During the soma ceremony's internal "ritual art" there is a gathering and ascent of the dispersed light into unity within that is reminiscent of Neoplatonic philosophy: "Endeavor to ascend into thyself, gathering in from the body all thy members which have been dispersed and scattered into multiplicity from that unity which once abounded in the greatness of its power. Bring together and unify the inborn ideas and try to articulate those that are confused and to draw into light those that are obscured."[21]

As we have shown, Eastern sources had an important impact upon early Greek thought. The Neoplatonists themselves claimed an Eastern origin for their ideas as well as those of Pythagoras and Plato. Pliny, Olympiodorus, Lactantius, and Clement of Alexandria all maintained that Plato both studied and was influenced by, and even plagiarized information from, the magi.[22] According to R. T. Wallis, "It seems certain that only Indian thought bears sufficient resemblance to Plotinus' introspective mysticism to be taken seriously as a possible source."[23]

There have been numerous studies of the correspondences between Neoplatonism and Indian philosophy.[24] None of these studies, however, is completely satisfactory. A deeper understanding of Indian philosophy, of the fundamental ideas contained within the Ṛg Veda, Atharva Veda, Āraṇykas, Brāhmaṇas, and twelve earliest Upaniṣads, is needed before a thorough comparison with Neoplatonic doctrines can be made.

Some of the most important correlations between soma and the soma ceremony can be seen in Neoplatonic theurgy, which is really a form of yoga. Since the Ṛg Vedic soma ceremony is the origin of the concept of the development of an interior subtle body of light, we can find many direct correlations between the rituals of Neoplatonic theurgy and the soma ceremony. That the astral or subtle body of the Neoplatonists had an Eastern origin was expressed by the Neoplatonist Numenius.[25]

Both Neoplatonism and the Ṛg Vedic soma ceremony share the belief that the physical body is an image of the state and functional ability of the soul or luminous essential nature. One's essential nature is expressed either fully or to a lesser extent according to the layering of impressions that fill the cave of the heart with darkness or light.

The physical body's prototypical design is derived from formless archetypes within the universal matrix of being. These archetypes are formed according to previous accumulations of sensual impressions layered in or over the light of the soul, which forces their activity to be expressed instead of one's original, luminous nature. Thus the physical body was anciently thought of as nothing more than the expressed nature of past thinking as deposited "subliminal activators," this being the origin of the concept of the Hindu notion of *karma*.

An important part of the soma ceremony ritual is performed to effect a removal and total displacement of these subliminal activators with pure, entheogenic, soma life-energy, reorienting a person through a reidentification process that becomes permanent. One forms a pneumatic energy body as the ground of one's being, which frees the essential nature or the soul so it can function in a pure state while still inside a physical body. These same ideas are found in Neoplatonic theurgy concerning the purification of the subtle or astral body.

The Indian influence upon Neoplatonism most likely came from the earliest Upaniṣads, which were themselves based upon the internalization of the Ṛg Vedic soma ceremony. In theurgy, as in both the soma ceremony and the early Upaniṣads, the subtle body is connected to the sun and the rays of the sun. As in India, the Neoplatonic subtle body is a vehicle used for ascension to the sun or realm of light. Also, the purification of the channels of this subtle body is what allows it to be separated from the physical body. Porphyry's view of theurgy was that it could purify the soul's pneumatic envelope; in other words, it could remove the sense impressions that hide the light of one's essential nature.[26] The seven cognitive sense-channels layer false impressions around the soul, and this is the source of the impurities. These impressions must be removed through a purification process. The soma ceremony purifies these channels through the ritualized influx of soma light-energy from the sun, which displaces incoming sense data to fashion a new body out of pure luminous energy. A similar process takes place in theurgy when one connects to the energy channels of the sun. Once the channels are purified, then the immortal vehicle, or golden ship, as it is called in the Atharva Veda, can leave the physical body.[27] The Neoplatonists used entheogens in their theurgic practices to induce interior light phenomena.[28]

The purification of the subtle body is accomplished through breath control and breathing practices, and the correspondences between the breathing practices of Neoplatonic theurgy and Indian yoga have recently been shown.[29] Such breathing practices were developed in the Ṛg Veda and the Atharva Veda. The pneumatic nature of the subtle body of light involves breath control practices using the logos and phonemes.

There is little doubt that the author or authors of the Chaldean Oracles, on which most of Neoplatonic theurgy is based, were working with texts of Indian origin, most probably the early Upaniṣads. They may have also been in contact with Indian sages with direct knowledge of yoga practices.[30]

A special form of inner devotional love within the heart of being is the entrance to the portal of light. The soul's return to its source is completely motivated in the Ṛg Vedic soma ceremony by the concept of devotional love within the heart. This love is a type of inner ecstasy that must be experienced to be understood. The part played by love in the soul's return is an important aspect of Plotinus's Neoplatonism. For Plotinus, love is more perfect when it does not aim at procreation, since such an aim indicates dissatisfaction with one's present condition. The love that Plotinus speaks of is a joyful, and seemingly solitary, contemplative love of the individual soul for its merging with the original unity.[31] The notions of duality do not arise in this state of being, which is unending bliss, consciousness, and oneness.

SOMA, GNOSTICISM, AND HERMETICISM

The presence of Indian sages in Greece and Egypt during the formulation of Gnostic, Hermetic, Neoplatonic, and alchemical schools has recently been shown in detail by Zacharias Thundy and Jean Sedlar.[32] In addition to early Indian influences from the Ṛg Veda and Upaniṣads, borrowings from Buddhist doctrines and stories also influenced Gnostic schools and Christianity. Indian influence, particularly Buddhist, on the development of Gnosticism, the New Testament, the Apocryphal Gospels, and Christian legend and lore has been well documented by Edward Conze, Jean Sedlar, and Richard Garbe.[33]

There are so many correspondences between the soma ceremony of the Ṛg Veda and the doctrines of the Gnostic and Hermetic texts that only a few of them can be discussed here, and the reader is referred to the references given in the notes for more information. I might add that because the original ideas of Indian philosophy found in its earliest texts, and the routes of influences to the West, are just beginning to be known, this research has only just begun. As the various texts and archaeological data are analyzed, more influences will become apparent.

Here I can discuss only two major concepts found in Gnostic and Hermetic texts that are important components of the Ṛg Vedic soma ceremony, with the Ṛg Veda remaining the oldest written source for these two concepts in their fully developed form. The first, a dominant part of the Ṛg Veda, is the "logos doctrine." In the Ṛg Veda the logos is called *vāc,* or the word. The second is the idea of the divine body of light. This notion of the "Primal Man" as the Anthropos, "Adamas, or Christ of light,"[34] is purely of Indo-Iranian origin but shows its first developed appearance in the the Indo-Aryan Puruṣa-Sūkta hymn of the Ṛg Veda (RV 10.90). This hymn is not a later addition but a formulation of the oldest ritual parts of the corpus. The hymn describes the basic solar cosmogony in the soma ceremony. It is directly connected to the cosmic pillar/axis nature of various deities and the "solar operations" performed during the ceremony. In the Ṛg Veda, as well as the Hermetic Poimandres and the Gnostic schools, the knowledge of the primal man of light is a central secret; according to the branch of the Valentinians, the primal cosmic man, or precosmic god within man, is the greatest and most hidden secret of the world, the key to immortality and salvation.

SOMA AND THE ORIGIN OF THE PRIMAL MAN OF LIGHT AS ANTHROPOS

Scholars earlier in the twentieth century tried to show the derivation of the Gnostic and Hermetic Anthropos from an Iranian source found in the Bundahishn. They had searched out Iranian, Babylonian, and Jewish elements to try to find the source for the Anthropos idea. They finally came to the conclusion that the Iranian Bundahishn myth of Gayomart's dismemberment was its most ancient developed form.[35] It was soon realized, however, that not only was the myth of Gayomart of a later date, but it did not contain the proper elements for the origins of the Anthropos idea as expressed in Gnostic and Hermetic texts. It was R. C. Zaehner who first pointed out that the precursor of the Iranian Gayomart myth came from the Indo-Aryan Ṛg Vedic myth of the Puruṣa-Sūkta.[36] The Puruṣa-Sūkta is an internalized pneumatic creation whose original primal form is androgynous. It is responsible for the creation of both the macrocosm and the microcosm or subtle body.

The Anthropos idea was passed on to the religions of Mesopotamia and later incorporated into Neoplatonism, alchemy, Islam, Judaism, Gnosticism, Christianity, and Hermeticism from Syria and other countries influenced by the Indo-Aryan Kassites, Hurrians, Hyksos, and Mitanni.[37] In a number of Gnostic systems the Anthropos is considered the fountainhead of a material—yet spiritual—principle indwelling in mankind and the world. This principle is variously defined as the soul, the pneuma, reason, or indeed as a combination of soul and pneuma or soul and mind. This is exactly how it is described in the Ṛg Vedic soma ceremony, where during the ritual the mind and senses are withdrawn within the heart of being. The concept of the pneuma can be traced in Greece from the pre-Socratic philosopher Anaximenes (500 B.C.E.), who was a student of Anaximander (547 B.C.E.), down to the Stoics. The idea refers not just to breath, but to a cosmic force. West has shown Indo-Iranian influences upon the thought of both Anaximander and Anaximenes, including a clear influence from Indian sources on Anaximenes' idea of "aer" or air as breath or pneuma. West traced these influences from Indian sources beginning with the Atharva Veda and the Upaniṣads. We can also add the Ṛg Veda soma ceremony, which used pneumatic stellar and solar magic in its rituals.[38]

In the Gnostic systems, where technical terminology has been evolved, the Anthropos is referred to by the name Jesus Patibilis, Inner Man, Son of Man, and Adakas. The ultimate origin of this concept is a problem of great intricacy, the solution of which has been very difficult to find. One reason is that any one scholar would have to master a wide variety of religious texts; another is that this issue is inextricably bound up with the problem of the origin of the "drama of the soul," that is, the problem of what the soul is, why the soul is the way that it is, why it needs liberation, and how it finds liberation. These mechanisms are difficult to trace and understand. The earliest record we have of human beings gaining immortality is in the Ṛg Veda. Therefore it is logical to look in there to find out what the concept of the soul is, and how immortality was obtained. This would answer the question of the origin of the soul drama; this problem has remained unsolved until now, that is, until the reconstruction of the Ṛg Vedic soma ceremony.

Many cultures of the ancient world believed that man has within him a divine element, a spark from the fire of the gods. In the Ṛg Veda this original spark was the luminous soma life-energy, dispersed as the souls of the world from the heaven world of light at the dawn of creation. In one tradition the original soma light is dispersed and diluted each time a human reproduces, decreasing the light and increasing matter. In another, souls as soma are continually flowing along invisible light rays for incarnation into human bodies.

Appearing under many names, but predominantly that of "soul," this original light was more than the sum of a person's subjective processes: it was a substance that came from God and returned to him.[39] This is the basic concept of the soul as Anthropos in the Gnostic schools and also in the Ṛg Vedic soma ceremony.

The idea of a primal man[40] of light who becomes the universe that is found in Gnostic and Hermetic texts is primarily associated in the Ṛg Veda with the development of the golden embryo. The Puruṣa-Sūkta hymn, which outlines the doctrine of the primal man or Anthropos, is derived from the fundamental cosmology of the oldest portions of the Ṛg Veda and the soma ceremony.

The ideas in the Puruṣa-Sūkta hymn derive from the myths of the Pole Star as cosmic tree/pillar and the midday sun as cosmic tree/pillar. The inner primal man of light or Anthropos is directly associated with this cosmic tree/pillar that derives from the golden embryo that develops within the central heart-sun. The heart-sun is placed or generated between the earth and the formless world of light, binding them together, and it is connected to the central cosmic-axis nature of many important Ṛg Vedic deities such as Indra, Varuṇa, Mitra, Agni, and, of course, Soma.

The Puruṣa-Sūkta hymn was derived from Indra's anthropocosmic body being identified as the golden embryo within the cosmic waters of the heart. This is one of the oldest themes of the Ṛg Veda, and it is associated directly with the creation of the universe, when a radiant column of light is placed between the unmanifest and manifest creation. It directly involves the origin and dispersion of soma light through the sun; in addition, the process of visualizing the generation of the golden embryo as the golden soma stalk within the heart appears in many of the older hymns of the Ṛg Veda related to the Anthropos. The soma stalk, like Indra, is seen as the cosmic pillar at the center of the universe, the axis mundi, and the Anthropos. "[Soma] the far-extended skambha [pillar], the adorned support of the sky, the filled-full amsüh [stalk] that encompasses everything. That [soma stalk] connects the two great world halves, [earth and heaven]. The kavi [poet] holds together the united pair [in his heart] and [partakes within] the refreshing food soma."[41] Other hymns say that this same soma stalk is the cosmic pillar or Anthropos within the heart of the priest. The soma plant as the cosmic Anthropos of light also goes through a dismemberment and rememberment cycle during the soma ceremony when it passes through the sun and then back again. These ideas about the Puruṣa-Sūkta as the primal man of light and the soul form the oldest myths of the Ṛg Veda.

The Sanskrit word *puruṣa* means "person," "soul," or "essential nature"; it is the arcane form that is immortal within us. The *puruṣa*, or soul, is a vast, subtle nature that lies beneath physical matter, binding it all together into a single whole as the primal man of light. Each soul or light spark is connected to the whole and has access to the whole. We can be one or many; our nature is not limited. The *puruṣa* as soul and soma is the divine spark that is hidden in matter and in our physical bodies. It is the hidden basis of layered, material creation. It is a cosmic luminous continuum, a column of brilliant light hidden within everyone, and it must be expressed if one is to attain final immortality. The soma ceremony is a procedure to express the Anthropos as the gathering of soma essences for the purpose of rememberment of the scattered soma light dispersed during creation. Because the Anthropos is man's real form, as well as the foundation of creation, the Puruṣa-Sūkta hymn states that man is everything that was in the past or that will be in the future.[42]

The Puruṣa-Sūkta hymn was derived from, and combined within, the soma ceremony and the interior practice of the expression of the golden embryo.

The twin Aśvins and the Greek Dioscuri both play important roles in the Ṛg Veda and Greek mysteries. In the Ṛg Veda, the Aśvins are divine physicians who are explicitly implored to give birth to and control the development of the interior golden embryo (egg) into the Anthropos. In the Greek tradition, the Dioscuri perform the same function as the Aśvins. The whole mystery of origin and destiny was said to be concealed in the symbolism of a radiant golden egg (embryo) suspended from the dome of the temple of the Dioscuri in Lakonia, near Sparta. It was said that those who understood this mystery had risen above all temporal limitations.

In the Ṛg Veda, the Aśvins control the alchemical transmutation of the white celestial soma into the golden entheogenic soma drink through the union of sun and moon lotus plants, personified as fire and water. This drink induces the birth and development of the interior entheogenic light as the luminous embryo-Anthropos located within the heart of the priest. A hymn in the Ṛg Veda describes the development of this light within the heart that allows the priest, after consuming soma, to move beyond his physical body through the agency of an anthropocosmic subtle body:

> Far beyond soar my ears, far beyond my eyes,
>
> Far away to this light which is set in my heart!
>
> Far beyond wanders my mind, its spirit [goes] to remote distances.[43]

The Anthropos as revealed in the Ṛg Vedic soma ceremony is apparently the original source of the knowledge of an arcane subtle body that the first man, Adam or Manu, had. This is the miracle body that is used to produce paranormal abilities, heal the sick, and rejuvenate the physical body.

The Ṛg Vedic Anthropos has had a profound influence on some of the most important ideas of later religious doctrine, some of which can be mentioned here. In the Gnostic Gospel of Thomas and the Corpus Hermeticum (8.2), for example, we find the concept of the self-generated light.[44] Just as in the Ṛg Vedic soma ceremony, the Gospel of Thomas talks about the mythology of the separation of the original unity and its return through the agency of the luminous subtle body. This luminous subtle-body form is the original body that Adam had before being wrapped up in matter after the Fall. According to logion 84 from the Gospel of Thomas, each person has a heavenly eternal image that came into existence before the human body. Furthermore, this divine image is normally concealed from the person and is awakened through ecstasy by either entheogens or devotion. Once awakened, this form unites one's true self to its heavenly origin. This is the same idea mentioned in 1 Corinthians 15:35–49, where Paul mentions two types of bodies, the earthly and the heavenly.[45] The immortal heavenly body is the subtle body of light as the Anthropos.

The apostle Paul both spoke of and practiced pneumatology. He believed the heavenly Adam as the primal Anthropos resided in every person as the pneumatic body of Christ as the Redeemer.[46] In 2 Corinthians 12:2–4, Paul mentions a man, who was apparently Paul himself, who identified himself with the Christ within as the Anthropos, and who was caught up to the third heaven, the abode of paradise. This type of ascent, by becoming identified with the inner cosmic Christ as Anthropos, has a specific pagan background. It is a type of ecstatic ascent through an anthropocosmic body that is generated within the heart by baptism with the celestial "water of life" (soma). This ecstatic ascent is different from the primitive shamanic one, and it is directly associated with Indo-Iranian magical forms of herbal mysticism. Paul infers that magical baptism is associated with secret teachings and rites performed by Jesus and is connected to a type of garment mysticism that produces the inner Anthropos. Paul's interpretation of mystical baptism as a means of ascent could have come from his contact with Mithraism in Tarsus, a site known to have Mithraic followers.[47] In Mandaean Gnosticism, the Anthropos is also the primordial man, called *adam kasia* or *adakas*, and is known as the secret Adam within each person. He has a body of light and the entire universe is derived from his pillarlike, anthropocosmic body, just as in the Ṛg Vedic Puruṣa-Sūkta. Upon identifying with the inner *adam kasia* or subtle body of light, a person gains immortality and ascends to his or her origin as a being of light.[48]

In Manichaean Gnosticism, the doctrine of the "radiant column of glory" that is used for ascension to the world of light is derived from Ṛg Vedic Anthropos ideas. This pillar of light is both a deity and a path by which liberated souls ascend to paradise.[49] The idea of the dispersion and the gathering of the heavenly light is a basic feature of the soma ceremony and is found in various Gnostic schools including Manichaeism. It is also the origin of the early Upaniṣadic doctrine of the gathering of the pneuma or *prāṇas* in Indian religion. This dispersion and gathering is also clearly established in the Atharva Veda, especially the Vrātya hymns. The ideas presented in these Indian texts is so similar to the ideas in Gnostic and Hermetic texts and Neoplatonism that it is easy to see that the early Indian texts are the probable original sources for them. Another example of these same ideas can be seen in the Gnostic Gospel of Philip and in the Gnostic Gospel of Eve as preserved by Epiphanius. For example,

> I am thou and thou art I, and where thou art I am, and in all things am I dispersed. And from wherever thou willst thou gatherest me; but in gathering me thou gatherest thyself. . . . This self-gathering is regarded as proceeding "pari passu" with the progress of "knowledge," and its completion as a condition for the ultimate release from the world. . . . He who attains to this gnosis and gathers himself from the cosmos. . . is no longer detained here but rises above the Archons . . . and by proclaiming this very feat the ascending soul answers the challenge of the celestial gatekeepers. . . . I have come to know myself and have gathered myself from everywhere.[50]

Not only did the Gnostics speak of the eternal pneumatic subtle body as Anthropos, but this pneumatic body was directly associated with the divine "water of life." The "water of life" is a type of celestial baptism for the pneumatic or perfected man who partakes of this "water of life" when identifying with the Anthropos within. In the Gnostic texts, this "water of life" is located above the firmament or created cosmos, just as soma is in the Ṛg Veda.[51] This is essentially an Indo-Aryan conception associated directly with soma as the "water of eternal life" that resides in the third heaven above the firmament and that is the goal not only of the Gnostic, but also of the soma priest, who, after consuming the entheogenic soma drink, is transported above this world to the abode of soma. The abode of soma is an immortal paradise where he drinks the celestial soma of immortality just like the gods. The same notion is found in Romans 7:22, 1 Corinthians 6:14, and Ephesians 3:16, 30, where Paul distinguishes between the physical body and the hidden inner spiritual body. This body is neither subject to the limits of space nor perceptible to our senses. Being the same as the subtle body developed in the soma ceremony, it is capable of union with the glorified body of Christ as Anthropos within the heart. The method of awakening this inner body is through a baptism of light, ritually portrayed by water baptism. Both light and water are essentially the same in the Ṛg Veda. Water is simply a more solidified or denser form of light. They both have heavenly origins. In the soma ceremony, the priest becomes bathed in heavenly soma in a type of baptism, which is part of the development of the Anthropos within the heart.

In the Jewish mystical tradition, the origin of the Merkabah or the "throne of God" is directly connected to the expression of a subtle luminous form within the heart, an idea similar to the Anthropos. The Jewish Merkabah as a generation of an interior subtle body of light has its probable origin in the Ṛg Vedic soma ceremony. This subtle form, called the "throne of glory," is connected to the Tree of Life and Paradise, is developed within the heart, and is the source of immortality and all magical practices within Judaism.[52] The word *merkabah* can also be translated as "chariot-throne," simultaneously a chariot and the throne of God. The *merkabah* is the fiery solar heart, which as the inner sun-chariot carries one's soul to God, and actually is God. It is directly associated with the Aśvins' entheogenic flower chariot drink that induces visionary light within the heart of the *somapa*. During the soma ceremony this entheogenic light is the inner pneumatic sun that rises up out of the body like a luminous or fiery chariot ascending toward the sky at dawn with the rising sun to the center of heaven. The relationship between Merkabah mysticism and the Hermetic and Gnostic ideas of the "man of light" or Anthropos have been discussed by Gershom Scholem.[53] In certain kabbalistic schools, the Merkabah mystics substituted the divine throne for the Gnostic Pleroma, a further correlation with the Anthropos idea. It is by the Merkabah and Pleroma that the mystic ascends to the realm of light.[54]

The same ideas are found in the concept of the throne of God in Islamic mysticism.[55] In the Islamic Sufi traditions, the Ṛg Vedic Anthropos idea has had a profound impact. The idea of "a man of light" or "Imam" within is described as a cosmic pillar of light and the foundation of the universe. The Imam as cosmic column of light is directly associated with both the Pole Star and the sun. In the Sufi tradition, the Imam is located as the divine light within the heart. Originally all of this came from the soma ceremony, but much of it was dispersed to other cultures through the earliest Upaniṣads. Although the Imam ideas have Zoroastrian correlations, the majority of the ideas that make up the Imam concept are derived from Indian sources. It is through the Imam that all of the miraculous paranormal powers are developed within Islamic tradition. As Amir-Moezzi has shown, the entire concept of the Imam cannot be understood unless viewed through Indian Sanskrit sources.[56]

In Christian doctrine, the glorified body of Christ, his ascension body, his body of eternity, is directly related to the Anthropos and subtle body within. This is the immortal body. This same type of body is connected to soma energy and the pneuma, or subtle breath energy, which is directly related to the Christian concept of the Holy Spirit.[57] It is through the aid of the Holy Spirit that one identifies with the subtle body of light as Jesus, the intermediary between the manifest and unmanifest worlds. The activation of the pneuma or Holy Spirit is through the power of the Word or Logos.

The Indian idea of cosmic man is also found in Greco-Egyptian alchemy. Zosimos, a Greco-Egyptian alchemist who lived around 300 C.E., employed these same ideas in the concept of the recovery of the original body of light that Adam had before his fall into matter. This is the main concern of Zosimos's work *On the Letter Omega.*[58] In addition, Zosimos asserts that the prime secret of the alchemical art was identical with the most hidden mystery of Mithraism.[59] Mary Boyce, a leading authority on Mithras, says that the Western Mithras tradition is not of Iranian origin; rather, its elements are of Indo-Aryan origin and can be found in the Ṛg Veda. The earliest known Mithraic temple, which was excavated at Atchana in northern Syria, dates back to 1500 B.C.E. (or before), and was associated with the Indo-Aryan Mitanni rather than the Iranians. It is known that entheogens were used in Mithraic rituals.[60] The Anthropos of light or the subtle body is a basic feature of the mysteries of Mithras. This same subtle body is also the basis of spiritual alchemy as mentioned by Zosimos.

The Corpus Hermeticum contains many conceptual and linguistic parallels with the Ṛg Veda and the Upaniṣads. India is actually mentioned a number of times in the texts; for example, when talking about paranormal abilities of the soul (tractate 11.19), India in particular is mentioned as if that were the land and source of the knowledge of miracles. The Asclepius (section 24) mentions Indians living in Egypt. There is little doubt that the writers of the Corpus had knowledge of the content of both Brahmanical and Buddhist scriptures. In the Poimandres (1.12–15), the motif of the cosmic man as Anthropos appears, although in a Hellenistic version. In verse 14, the cosmological structure of the world of light is inverted with respect to the world of matter. This is represented as a reflection in the water (primal waters of creation).[61] The primal man of light, during his descent from the realm of light, becomes wrapped up in matter, which, as verse 15 says, makes humankind, of which the Anthropos is the prototype. Human beings thus have a material body, which hides within it the original light as the primal Anthropos. Upon re-identification with the inner Anthropos of light, human beings can ascend back to their immortal origins. One of the most important points made in the Poimandres is that the body of light contains the energies of the governors. These are the seven demiurges that are also associated with the Anthropos in the soma ceremony.

In the Ṛg Vedic soma ceremony the Anthropos is generated within the heart of being. The spherical soul as the heart-sun or Anthropos is also a star body and is found both in Gnostic schools and in alchemy. The star body or soul usually has seven projections, which correspond to the seven cognitive sense channels of the head. Speech or logos is sometimes considered an eighth projection. Both of these concepts are found in the Ṛg Vedic soma ceremony.

The primordial man of light or Anthropos as presented in the Ṛg Vedic soma ceremony is as small as a seed, yet invisibly coextensive with the entire cosmos. From this seed a great pneumatic tree of light, the soma tree, is generated within the heart of being. It is clearly specified in the soma ceremony that the subtle Anthropos of light related to the cosmic pillar/tree extends its rays as branches to touch all creation. Therefore, it is the interior Anthropos that allows mortal man to become immortal as well as to become the creator of the universe. In the Ṛg Vedic soma ceremony, the process of expression of the interior light is initiated by *vāc* or the Logos.

The Soma Ceremony and the Origin of the Logos

The Word or Logos is identified with the Anthropos in the soma ceremony and is not separate from it. This is also true for the Gnostic and Hermetic schools, as shown by Carl Kraeling,

> The Gnostic Anthropos is none other than this large or great Man, the personification of the cosmic Logos, says Leisegang. As a matter of fact that is exactly what the supreme Anthropos does in the Christian strata of the Naasene document. Shorn of his cosmic content the same Logos is associated with the Anthropos, as we have seen, in the system of Valentinus, as his father, and in the Poimandres as his brother, while in the Gospel of Mary, the Man is none other than the sum of Nous and Ennoia, whose manifestation the cosmic Logos represents.[62]

In the Ṛg Vedic soma ceremony, and during the origin of the creation of the universe, the divine Logos was separated from its divine unity. It was separated into the higher unuttered and unactivated logos of the supernal world and the uttered and spoken logos that is the speech of mankind, which is connected to the manifested cosmos. This idea is the probable origin of the pattern of the logos concepts in Gnosticism, Neoplatonism, and Hermeticism. This same pattern is used or is related to the dispersion or dismemberment and the absorption or rememberment motif of the universal word/light. The activation within the heart of being for the reunification of the logoi is initiated by secret syllables. When this takes place during the soma ceremony the logos is related to the fiery breath as a mixture of fire and pneuma, which is closely related to the Greek concept of the logos. The logos is what binds together the separated parts.

We would expect that the origin of the logos idea would be developed by a priesthood who had composed a special liturgical language with a potent magical grammar. The earliest such language that was specifically developed for the alteration of consciousness and used for ascension is found in Indo-Aryan Vedic Sanskrit. This language may go back to 4000 B.C.E., with its roots in the earliest beginnings of Indo-Iranian language. Its modification into a specific magical language probably took place between 3000 and 2200 B.C.E.

The Word as God and the supreme self is the fundamental basis of all Ṛg Vedic hymnal compositions, as well as the priestly version of Vedic Sanskrit itself. The logos doctrine can be traced back in Greek philosophy to its alleged source in Heraclitus, who received this idea from Indo-Iranian sources.[63] It has also been thought that the origin of the idea of the logos may have originated in the Egyptian Memphite creation myth, which has been dated to approximately 500 B.C.E.[64] However, in the Memphite creation myth, the concept of the logos in creation is not developed fully enough to have been the source for the logos ideas. In addition, the Memphite myth of creating by the logos in combination with the heart appears to be an influence upon Egyptian religion from an outside source. Antecedents for this late creation myth in Egypt are vague. Even Egyptologists are uncertain as to the originality of the Memphite creation myth; most agree that it is from a later period.[65] As noted previously, we know that Egypt had close contact with Indo-Aryans at least since the middle of the second millennium B.C.E., and we also know there was an Indian colony established as early as 500 B.C.E. in Memphis, where they have found Indian-made votive offerings to the god Ptah. It is not too hard to see an Indo-Aryan influence on this late Egyptian creation myth, especially when the fundamental basis of the Ṛg Vedic soma ceremony is creation by the logos through the heart.

In the Gnostic and Hermetic texts, the logos is connected to light and the generation of light. It is used as a fiery breath (pneuma) to stir up the elements in creation. The logos, just as in the soma ceremony, is used to bring forth seven deities who are related to destiny and the seven sensory openings. The logos is also split up between the created cosmos and the uncreated origin. The Greek word *logos* is derived from the root *leg*, meaning "to gather." This same notion is in the Ṛg Vedic soma ceremony, where fire gathers everything together. By pronouncing the word internally within the heart, a fiery breath is generated. This begins the process of the gathering together within the heart of the dispersed soma light particles to form or express the subtle body as Anthropos. The chanting of hymns, as in the soma ceremony, produces a musical quality that aids in the expression of the subtle body through the seven sensory channels. These seven channels were also seen as layers or spheres around the soul. They were sometimes equated with the seven planets. Thus, we have the origin of the influence of the music of the spheres on the soul, associated originally with the rhythmical chanting meters of the soma hymns.

The Greeks probably obtained their knowledge of the logos from Indian sources in the early Ṛg Veda and the later Upaniṣads. The Greeks then transmitted their knowledge of the logos to the developing Gnostic and Hermetic literature. The logos doctrine in the Christian Gospel of John (1:3–4) is closely related to the logos idea in the Ṛg Veda: In the beginning was the word and the word was God.[66] Compare the logos ideas presented above from the soma ceremony to those found in the Gospel of John and the Gnostic schools.[67]

SOMA AND THE GNOSTIC/ALCHEMICAL STAR BODY

Through the inner processes of the Gnostic schools the physical body obtained an internal spiritualized form of light. In Gnostic circles, this body of light was called the radiant rayed body or starlike body, because its appearance is like a point of light with seven projected rays. The star body is also mentioned by the Neoplatonic philosopher Hierocles (450 C.E.) and the Platonist Philoponus (650 C.E.), who said there is a "kind of body that is forever attached to the soul, of a celestial nature, and for this reason ever-lasting, which they call radiant *(augoeides)* or star-like *(astroeides).*"[68]

The star body was thought to reside within the head (Fig. 6) because the seven rays of the star body are the same as the seven sensory channels of the head. The star body, however, does not reside in the head, but in the heart, as is revealed in the Ṛg Veda, where it is said that the head and heart become sewn together during the soma ceremony. Thereafter the star body resides in the heart. This is the body by means of which union with God takes place and paranormal ability occurs. As has been mentioned, the earliest documented cases of human beings performing paranormal feats such as walking on water, levitation, psychogenic creation, and rejuvenation, as well as attaining immortality, come from the entheogenic soma tradition in the Ṛg Veda. The formation of the body of stars *(devapīlukāya)* by which one becomes a radiant *ṛṣi* in the soma tradition is fundamental in the attainment of magical abilities and the performance of miracles. The original source of knowledge of the subtle body of stars comes from the Ṛg Veda soma tradition. Marsilio Ficino was not wrong to attribute this body to the magi.[69] It is through the formation and use of this special body, which projects rays (invisible to sight), that the traditions of Persian, Neoplatonic, Hermetic, Arabic, and European magical traditions are derived. Through Arabic and Gnostic—but primarily Neoplatonic—sources, the Islamic philosopher al-Kindī (d. 873 C.E.) obtained information about the Ṛg Vedic star body and its use in magical practices through projection of its pneumatic rays. It is mainly through al-Kindī's book,

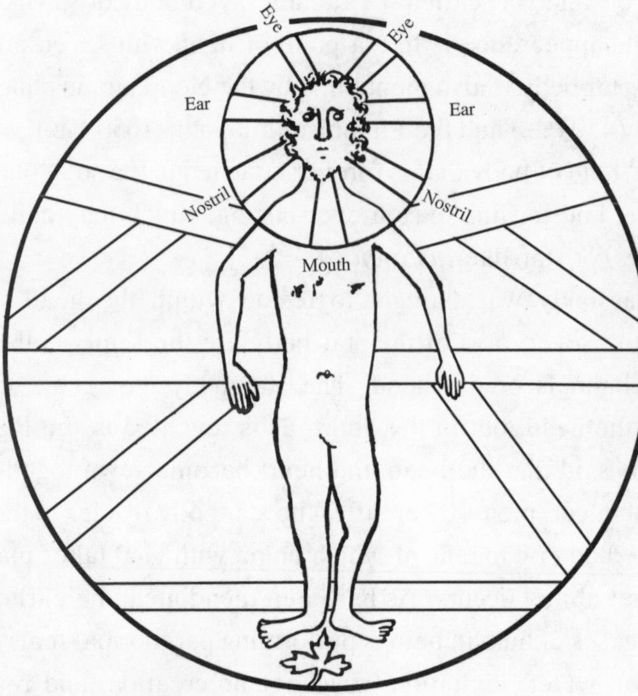

a.

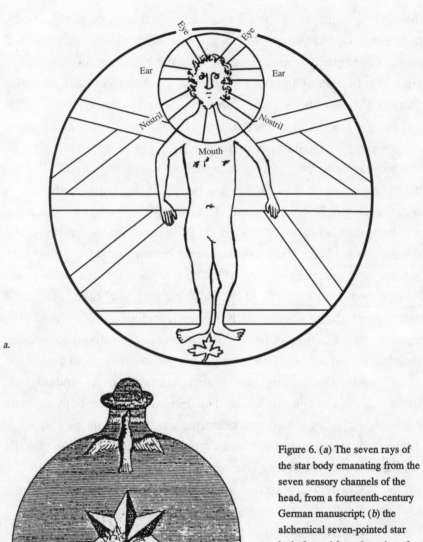

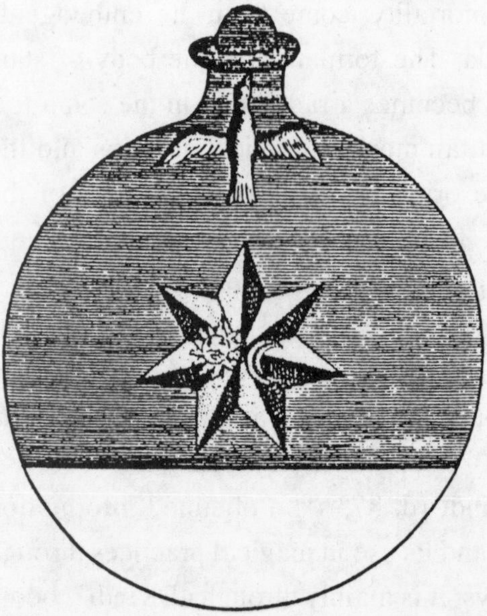

b.

Figure 6. (*a*) The seven rays of the star body emanating from the seven sensory channels of the head, from a fourteenth-century German manuscript; (*b*) the alchemical seven-pointed star body formed from the union of sun and moon within the hermetic vessel as the heart. The ascent of the soul is symbolized by a dove. From Barchusen's *Elementa Chemiae,* Leiden, 1718.

called *De radiis* or The Rays, that the Western magical traditions received their most important source for ancient Indo-Aryan pneumatic magic. Al-Kindī had a direct influence upon Roger Bacon, Marsilio Ficino, Giordano Bruno, and John Dee. Al-Kindī knew of only a portion of these magical processes that originated in the Ṛg Vedic soma ceremony. Through the correct ritual use of the entheogenic soma drinks, pneumatic magic is greatly enhanced.

We can awaken the body of stars, or rays, but, according to the Gnostic schools, to unite it with the deity depends upon the will of God. This unity is accomplished by the mystery of grace, achieved through devotion. This inner hidden spiritual body as conceived by the Gnostics was not subject to the limits of space, nor was it cognizable by the senses; it was the same as the glorified body of Christ. The formation of the body of stars or rays of which the Gnostics speak is brought about through a baptism of light. The origin of the notion of the baptism of light comes from the Ṛg Vedic soma ceremony, where this light is soma and is derived from the third heaven above the stars, which is soma's abode. According to the Ṛg Veda, it is this celestial soma that lights up the stars. Since the soul/Anthropos is composed of soma light, just as the stars, it is also called a star body; its shape also makes it look starlike.[70] This baptism of light is the same as that which occurs in the soma ceremony of the Ṛg Veda. The seven sensory channels become flooded by radiant, white, soma light-energy as they are absorbed back into the heart-soul to form the fiery pneumatic body. This downflow of celestial soma is the same as the baptism of the celestial "water of life" mentioned in various Gnostic texts.[71] The formation of the body of stars is described in the Gnostic Book of Jeu.[72] The star body is graphically shown in many European alchemical illustrations as the culmination of the whole work of alchemy connected with the philosophers' stone. It is usually depicted with seven projections coming from the human head, corresponding to the seven cognitive sense channels that get absorbed into the heart and then projected back outward through the same sensory channels. This same subtle form is developed within the heart of the priest taking part in the soma ceremony. Its development transmutes the priest into a *ṛṣi* and a *deva*, or "shining one"; in other words, he becomes a radiant star, and he is sometimes even identified with a star in the heavens.

7 SOMA AND EUROPEAN ALCHEMY

Knowledge of the alchemical procedures found in the Ṛg Vedic soma ceremony have been incorporated directly into European alchemical treatises, which accounts for many of the similarities found in Indian religion and European alchemy. Many of the different routes by which Indian cosmological ideas were passed on to Greek, Jewish, and Islamic philosophers have been discussed in chapter 6. These philosophers in turn influenced the writers of European alchemical texts. Before proceeding to discussions of European elixir theories, the philosophers' stone, and the alchemical structure of the soma ceremony, let us examine, in more detail, the symbols of the inverted tree and the seven-pointed star body.

Soma and Inverted-Tree Cosmology in Western Mystical Traditions

The symbol of the cosmic tree in both its upright and inverted forms is clearly found in the Ṛg Veda. Both forms of the cosmic tree are used as the basic formulation of the cosmogony and cosmology of the soma sacrifice. The inverted tree appears to be of Indo-Aryan and Harappan origin and has no other antecedents. The Indus Valley (Harappan) and the Indo-Aryan cultures developed in close connection with each other before the composition of the Ṛg Vedic hymns. The cosmic tree in its upright and inverted forms is found on Indus Valley seals as well as in the Ṛg Veda, and some of the seal impressions indicate that the religious beliefs of the Indus Valley culture are similar to those of the soma ceremony. The cosmic tree in both traditions was the fig tree. According to Simo Parpola, "The inverted tree is not derived from the Assyrian tree: its visualization as the fig tree [in the Ṛg Veda] links it with the Harappan sacred tree motif . . .," which suggests that the inverted tree derives from a combination of Indo-Aryan and Harappan beliefs.[1]

In the soma ceremony there are clear indications that the heavenly world, beyond our cosmos and from which soma or light originates, is inverted with respect to the manifest world of creation. This concept of the two mirrored worlds merging within the heart of the priest is a basic ritual component of the oldest books of the Ṛg Veda, and the foundation of the soma ceremony.

It appears that the cosmic tree had already been formulated into a divine ritual of the soma ceremony before the Indo-Aryans (Hurrian/Mitanni) entered northern Syria before 2000 B.C.E. The Indo-Aryans had already unified both the concept of the cosmic tree and cosmic pillar as well as the older cosmology of the Pole Star with the later solar cosmology. These ideas are well documented in the

Ṛg Veda in the union of Mitra (sun/day) with Varuṇa (Pole Star/night), forming the composite deity Indra, who personifies the cosmic pillar/tree of light that unites the two. This unification is accomplished through the twin Aśvins' ritual union of the sun (day) and moon (night) lotus plants that induce an entheogenic experience of luminous immortality.[2] Because of this unification, the early ritualized soma ceremony used a tree trunk with all its limbs removed, which made it look like a cosmic pillar. Because the soma ritual was designed to incorporate both the upright and inverted conceptions of the cosmic tree, no limbs could remain along its trunk; these would be superimposed during the ritual. The prominent cosmological features within later Assyrian religion are derived from the older Mitanni concept of the soma ceremony and the uniting of the cosmic pillar and cosmic tree motifs in both their upright and inverted forms. The early seal impressions of Mitanni influence show limbs superimposed upon the cosmic pillar. The Ṛg Vedic cosmic tree has six branches arranged in pairs along its trunk, with the trunk as the seventh branch. These seven branches correspond to the seven sensory pathways. The tree itself represents the cosmic pillar/tree as the subtle body.

In Ṛg Vedic cosmology, the unmanifest realm above is represented by an upright tree. The manifest world below is represented by an inverted tree. These can be graphically depicted as two triangles pointing in opposite directions and mirroring each other △▽. This is the probable origin of the graphic representation of two triangles opposed to each other found in European alchemical and magical traditions. The soma priest used fire along the cosmic pillar/tree to invert it, making it an upward-pointing triangle △. This initiated a reunification of the manifest and unmanifest worlds. The fire (Agni) is said in the Ṛg Veda to be born directly from the entheogenic lotus *(puṣkara)* that induces the inner fire in the heart. When the two triangles representing the manifest and the unmanifest worlds merge in the heart as explained in the Ṛg Vedic soma ceremony, the formation of the six-pointed star body of light results △▽=✡. Fire reverses the inverted tree of manifestation by uniting the manifest with the unmanifest, forming a union of opposites. At this stage celestial soma merges with terrestrial Agni and lights up the solar heart. The six-pointed star body is really a seven-pointed star body. Along the trunk there are three sets of pairs of limbs, which equal six points. The central pillar is itself the seventh point of the seven-pointed star body. The luminous solar body of light emerges from the primal waters of creation in the heart-ocean. This inner star body formed by the union of opposites is found at the basis of many Western mystical traditions including magic, Gnosticism, Kabbalah, alchemy, Hermetic traditions, and the works of Jacob Boehme, Robert Fludd, and John Dee.

The Indo-Aryan Mitanni passed on the cosmological idea of inversion to the Assyrians, who also developed a concept of the highest heaven and the material universe as being reflections of each other. We see this in the case of the Assyrian sun god, Assur, who emanated heaven as his primary manifestation to mirror his existence to the world.[3] The dramatic change in the presentation of the cosmic tree and pillar that the Mitanni symbolism introduced shows new cosmological ideas presented in Assyrian texts that are of probable Mitanni and Indo-European origin. This influence extended to all the countries of western Asia, the Near East, the Middle East, Crete, and Egypt.

In Egypt we find the concept of an inverted afterlife, where the kingdom of the dead was upside down in relation to that of the living.[4] This concept is the same as in the Ṛg Vedic soma ceremony: If the eye is not united to the sun, which begins the union of the unmanifest formless light with the manifest form of matter within the heart, then after death the deceased are plunged into primeval darkness and are unable to see the rays of the sun. Without this union of the manifest and unmanifest, the dead are placed in an inverted, dark world, unable to perceive the world of light because it is inverse to them. This conception is derived from Indo-Aryan cosmology as found in the Ṛg Vedic soma ceremony. The most recent archaeological findings at Hierakonpolis have shown that the founders of Egyptian civilization originated in Iran, which was part of a larger group of connnected civilizations that extended from the Persian Gulf to the Indus River in India.[5]

The source of the inverted-tree cosmology is found in the Ṛg Veda and is directly associated with soma and the soma ceremony, from which Indian religions derive the functional nature of the inverted cosmic tree. Here we are looking at the probable source of all the later mystical traditions that use the inverted cosmic-tree motif, including European alchemy.

The inverted cosmic tree represents the manifestation of the physical universe from its seed source in the sun or heaven, located at the cosmic center. The sun is located in the womb from which the material universe is downwardly created, like a human baby born headfirst. The subtle ascension body of light, as the luminous heart-soul, is inverted to its physical body. This is why in kabbalistic texts we find illustrations of the flaming or glowing upward-pointing spiritual heart of light inverted to its physical counterpart. When the person begins the process of return to the origin, he or she does not use the physical body, but the subtle body. In Indian yoga, the subtle body of light is inverted in relation to the physical body, and the subtle body of light of the cosmos is inverted in relation to its material forms. As mentioned in numerous Hindu yoga and tantric texts and explained correctly by Alain Daniélou, "Like the relation of the chrysalis to the butterfly, so the subtle body is inverted in regard to the gross body."[6] The subtle body remains inverted to the physical body until Agni as fire *(kuṇḍalinī)* reverses it. This whole process originated in the soma ceremony of the Ṛg Veda, in which an entheogenic herbal drink helped to induce this luminous reversal.

The inversion also represents the soteriological path back to divinity and out of the confinement of matter. Inversion is also represented in the withdrawal of the senses, a reversal of their normal outgoing function. We shall see later on, however, that the withdrawal of the senses and their re-projection paradoxically allow one to live in the physical cosmos of matter and still be united with God or essential nature.

The concept of the Indo-Aryan inverted tree is found among Lapp shamans, Islam, the Kabbalah, various European alchemical texts, and in the writings and illustrations of Robert Fludd, Jacob Boehme, and John Dee. The inverted tree is found even in Plato's *Timaeus:* "That part (soul) which we say dwells in the summit of our body and lifts us from earth towards our celestial affinity, like a plant whose roots are not in earth, but in the heavens."[7] It is this inverted inner divine power that keeps the physical body upright (Fig. 7).

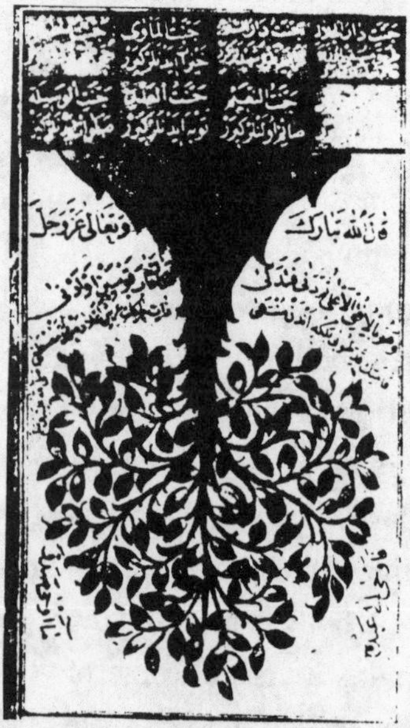

Figure 7. Inverted tree in Islam, from an eighteenth-century Turkish prayer book. By permission of the Trustees of the Chester Beatty library.

Indian ideas of soma and the cosmogonic reversable soma tree of the Ṛg Vedic soma ceremony had a significant impact upon the fundamental cosmology at the heart of Western esotericism. That Islam would incorporate the inverted-tree motif and other religious and philosophical texts shows the very high regard and respect it had for Indian religious philosophy. The inverted-tree cosmology found in the Ṛg and Atharva Vedas was incorporated into the later Indian literature of the Upaniṣads and from there was probably borrowed by Islam.

The Jewish Kabbalists read the Arabic works and used the concept of the inverted tree in their religious speculations. They also wrote alchemical works and incorporated the inverted tree as a major cosmogonic symbol directly related to the elixir as the philosophers' stone. It is also known from such texts as the *Shoshan Yesod Olam* that Kabbalists used entheogenic plants to induce visionary ecstatic states as in the soma ceremony.[8] The trunk of the cosmic tree was viewed in the same sense in Judaism as in the Ṛg Veda, that is, as a luminous pneumatic pillar that houses both God and one's soul as a spark of God. In Genesis (28:17–22) we find the Indo-Iranian conception of the cosmic pillar as the source and abode of God. "Jacob set up a pillar that was the house of God." Jacob remarks that the pillar is not only the "abode of God but the gateway to heaven." In kabbalistic books this pillar is associated with the primordial man of light as Anthropos, which is called Adam Kadmon and by which one performs miracles and ascends out of the body.[9] In kabbalistic texts such as the *Zohar* and *Bahir* we also find the inverted-tree cosmology and cosmogony.[10] The pillar-trunk of the inverted tree in both the *Zohar* and *Bahir* represents an internal experience like that found in the soma ceremony. This trunk is a luminous pneumatic pillar/tree that arises from the solar heart in both the microcosm (man) and the macrocosm (universe). The common pillar-trunk represents both the upright and inverted trees.[11] Another Indian belief commonly found in both the Kabbalah and in Hasidism that is associated with the inverted tree, by which souls descend to the earth, is the notion of reincarnation *(gilgul)*.[12] In the *Bahir* there is a direct mention of the trunk of the cosmic tree as a pillar that connects heaven to earth. It is by this pneumatic pillar that the enlightened, righteous, or perfected man (Anthropos) ascends to heaven. Scholem states that this kabbalistic idea is originally of Iranian origin. It would ultimately be derived from the *haoma*/soma ceremonies.[13] This idea probably came from either Arabic sources or directly from Indian Upaniṣadic sources that date back to around 900 B.C.E. It could also have come partly from Syrian and Assyrian sources that are ultimately derived from Indo-European Hurrian/Mitanni symbolism and cosmology, which the Mitanni introduced into northern Syria. The most likely sources, however, are the Arabic and Indian sources. Kabbalists probably would not have obtained these ideas directly from the Ṛg Veda, even though its hymns are their ultimate source.

The Jewish Kabbalists were in contact with various Indian writings, as we can see from reading their texts. Exactly which Indian writings is not completely clear, but it can be assumed that it was the Upaniṣads, which had been translated into Arabic, and maybe parts of other Hindu ritual texts. Another possibility is the Atharva Veda, which had been partly translated into Arabic with other Indian medical writings. Still another important source would have been Indians in the West who knew a great deal about yoga, as well as Indian ideas that passed to Jewish scholars through Sufism. In addition, the empire of the Medes, comprised of Iranians and Indo-Aryans, had a great influence upon Israel's religion when the former conquered Mesopotamia around 600–550 B.C.E., setting the Israelites free from Assyrian captivity. As a by-product of their release, Israel became closely aligned with the Medean-Persian empire and absorbed many Indo-Iranian doctrines into Judaism. These included certain cosmological ideas, fire worship, dualism (God/devil, future life as heaven and hell), the concept of angels, resurrection, and so on.[14]

An example of Indian yogic influence upon a Jewish kabbalistic writer appears in the writings of Abraham Abulafia, who was born in 1240 C.E. and founded what is called the ecstatic Kabbalah. Abulafia taught various breathing techniques combined with repetitions of divine names that have been described here as the logos doctrines. His techniques were based on Indian prototypes and show similarities with those of the soma ceremony. These techniques use sounds (logoi) to vibrate (in Sanskrit, *vipra*) and heat up (in Sanskrit, *tapas*) the spiritual heart area to form an upward-moving fiery pillar or tree of light. This heating is not exactly equivalent to actual heat; instead, it is a deep, ecstatic love felt in the spiritual heart, which feels like a warming inside. This heating automatically prepares the heart for the downwardly emanated influx of God as divine light or soma.[15]

In many European alchemical texts we find the inverted cosmic-tree motif. One of the many paradoxical qualities of the so-called, *arbor philosophica* is that it is said to grow upside down. Hence, it is called the *arbor inversa*, the inverted tree.[16] Contained within the *Mirror of Alchimy* by Roger Bacon is a Hebrew alchemical text translated into English in 1597 on the nature of the philosophers' stone and its birth. It says,

> Take it therefore and work it as the Philosopher has told you in his book, when he named it after this manner. Take a Stone which is not a Stone, that is neither a Stone nor of the nature of a Stone. It is a Stone whose mineral is generated in the summit of the mountains: and here by mountains, the Philosopher understandeth living creatures, whereupon he said. Son, go to the mountains of India, and to its caves, & pull

> out thence precious stones which will melt in the water when they are put into it. And this water is that which is taken from other mountains and hollow places. They are stones Son, and they are not stones, but we call them so for a similarity which they have to stones. And you must know, *that the roots of their minerals are in the air, and their tops in the earth.*[17]

This description of the stone that is not a stone actually refers to the philosophers' stone as an Indian plant. In this text the philosophers' stone is found in the mountain caves of India. This comes from the Ṛg Vedic conceptions that the philosophers' stone as soma is found upon the summit of the cosmic mountain. It is found in the cave of the heart where the cosmic mountain is located.

Other European alchemical treatises also speak of the inverted tree:

> It has the roots of its minerals above in the air and its branches below in the earth. Also in the *Gloria Mundi*, it is mentioned that the philosophers have said that the root of its minerals is in the air and its head in the earth. George Ripley describes the tree with its roots in the air and, elsewhere, as being rooted in the glorified earth, in the earth of paradise or in the future world.[18]

In European alchemical texts the movement of the luminous elixir through the cosmic tree as its sap that flows to all creation is the same as soma in the ancient Ṛg Vedic soma ceremony. The luminous fluid created by the nuptial union of opposites runs through the veins of the philosophical tree. This cosmic sap is of a subtle nature, and it saturates the bodies of the sun and moon while effecting their total fusion. It is described as an oily water, just as soma is sometimes described in the Ṛg Veda. It is the philosophical stone as a plant from which the branches of the luminous philosophical tree multiply into infinity.[19] The philosophers' tree shares with the stone the qualities of autonomy and universality (Fig. 8).

Commenting on the work of the Arabic alchemist known as Senior, the alchemical text *Consilium Coniugii* says,

> Thus the stone is perfected of and in itself. For it is the tree whose branches, leaves, flowers, and fruits come from it and through it and for it, and it is itself whole or the whole and nothing else. Another alchemical author says: Of itself, from, in, and through itself is made and perfected the stone of the wise. For it is one thing only: like a tree (says Senior), whose roots, stem, branches, twigs, leaves, flowers, and fruit are of it and through it and from it and on it, and all come from one seed. It is itself everything, and nothing else makes it.[20]

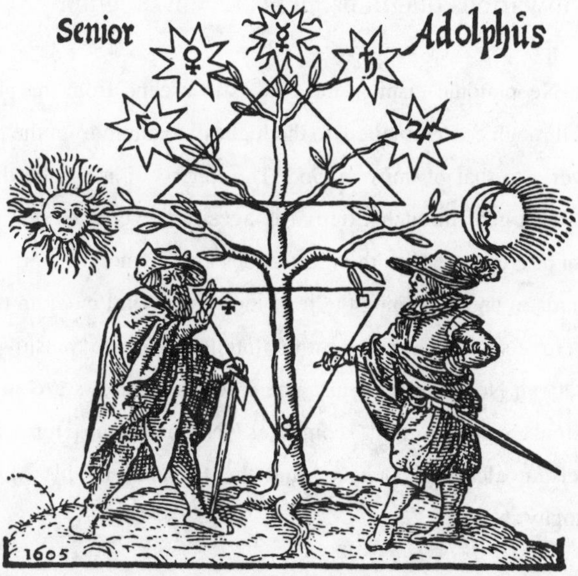

Figure 8. The cosmic tree of universal matter with seven branches and opposing triangles. From *Occulta Philosophia*, Frankfurt, 1613.

The European alchemist Gerhard Dorn summarizes the alchemists' ideas of their philosophical tree in the following manner: "On account of the likeness alone, and not substance, the philosophers compare their material to a golden tree with seven branches, thinking that it encloses in its seed the seven metals, and that these are hidden in it, for which reason they call it a living thing."[21]

We find the inverted-tree cosmology and the idea that the world of light is inverse to the material world in the cosmological and alchemical philosophy of the Hermeticist Robert Fludd (1574–1637), who based his entire cosmology unwittingly on the ancient Ṛg Vedic soma ceremony. He borrowed his cosmological system from various Christian, Gnostic, Neoplatonic, Hermetic, alchemical, and kabbalistic sources, which in turn had borrowed their systems from the Greeks or Arabs, who had borrowed them from India. William Huffman has clearly stated Fludd's basic cosmology, which Fludd illustrated in various diagrams, in his recent biography.

> In true Neoplatonic fashion, the goal is to ascend from the physical world, through contemplation, to the highest, to climb from the quadripart world to that of unity in God. The inner vision can be directed toward that goal through external images, to reverse as it were the process of creation. Thus the illustrations are far more important than mere aids to understanding the text; they are a vital medium that the imaginative soul uses to connect the Intellect with the Sensitive Soul, in Fluddean Neoplatonic terms. The whole structure is a completely consistent scheme that combines Neoplatonic Hermeticism, Paracelsian alchemy, Genesis, and the Cabala into his Mosaicall Philosophy.[22]

Most of Fludd's works are in Latin. But one major book, his *Mosaicall Philosophy*, is in English. Several other texts have been translated into English. There have also been several detailed English studies of his entire corpus. Fludd had detailed illustrations showing his cosmological system made for most of his books. From a careful observation of his cosmological diagrams we can clearly see correspondences with Indian cosmology. Some similarities include the inverted kabbalistic tree as the downward spiral of creation (Fig. 9a). The created universe of matter is shown as a mirror image of heaven. In his *Utriusque cosmi historia*, Fludd says that the cosmological structure of the universe is like upward and downward triangles (upright and inverted trees) that are mirrored through the medium of the "watery world"[23] (Fig. 9b). This image is identical to that in the Ṛg Veda, in which the primal waters that separate the heavenly world of light above from the manifested world of matter below act as a mirror, the medium of the cosmic waters in which the two worlds are inverted. We see the union of the world of light with dark matter as a union of opposites that creates the solar heart. Fludd shows the embryonic creation of the sun. Fludd's system contains the central sun as the solar heart, formed from two inverted triangles (Fig 9c). The seven *cakras* are shown aligned with the creation (Fig. 9d).

The cosmogonic idea of physical creation inverted with respect to heaven also appears in the work of Jacob Boehme (1575–1624).[24] In Boehme's work we find that the cosmic tree of the soul grows up from the heart of man and bears the fruit of immortality, just as the soma tree grows from the heart and gives immortality in the soma ceremony. As this tree grows upward, it destroys the world tree of matter and illusion. The central sun is the heart in Boehme's system as well. The concept of the manifest world of creation and the heaven of light being in inverse relation to each other is seen in many of the drawings of Johann Gichtel and Dionysius Andreas Freher, both pupils of Boehme's writings. Their diagrams also show the union of the manifest with the unmanifest as the union of opposites or oppos-

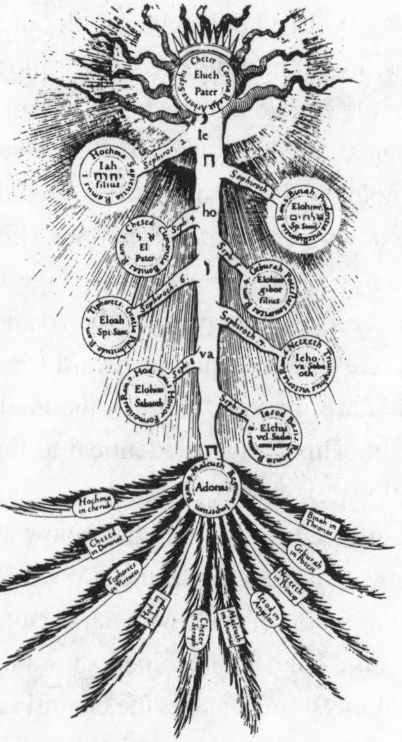

a.

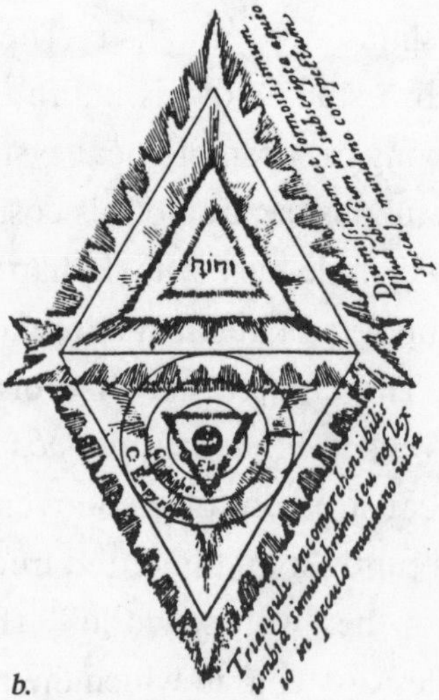

b.

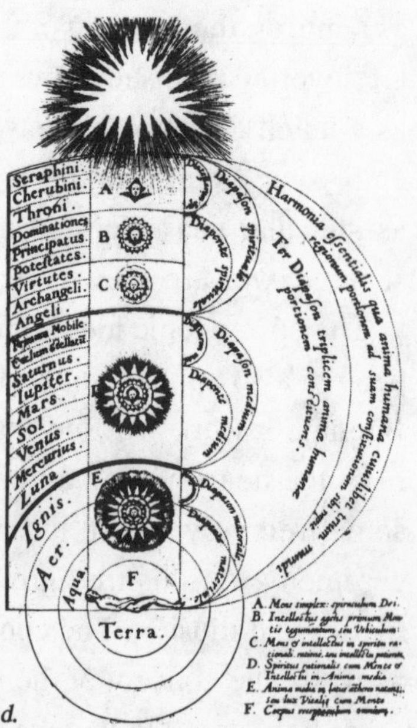

d.

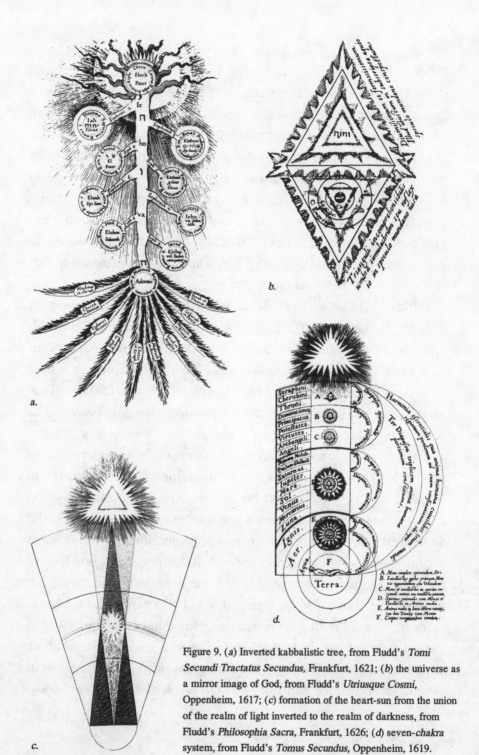

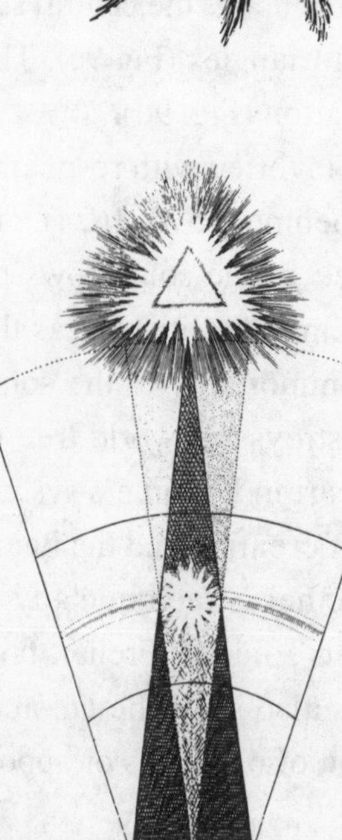

c.

Figure 9. (*a*) Inverted kabbalistic tree, from Fludd's *Tomi Secundi Tractatus Secundus,* Frankfurt, 1621; (*b*) the universe as a mirror image of God, from Fludd's *Utriusque Cosmi,* Oppenheim, 1617; (*c*) formation of the heart-sun from the union of the realm of light inverted to the realm of darkness, from Fludd's *Philosophia Sacra,* Frankfurt, 1626; (*d*) seven-*chakra* system, from Fludd's *Tomus Secundus,* Oppenheim, 1619.

ing triangles. The union takes place in the heart. As discussed previously, the Ṛg Vedic Puruṣa-Sūkta or primal man of light and cosmic pillar/tree is symbolically hermaphroditic, containing the restoration of all opposites in a perfect unity of being. In Boehme's mystical system, the androgyny or union of opposites as Christ is restored to perfection in the same fashion as in the soma ceremony and involves the same elements. The process takes place in the heart through devotional ecstasy and involves pneuma (divine air-spirit), Agni (fire), and Soma (as light and spiritual water or ambrosia). Boehme says,

> Christ cannot become manifest in man . . . [unless the soul feeds] upon the water-fountain, then the spirit of love . . . becomes fiery, and lays hold of the fire-root . . . [then] the soulish centre from the fire-nature is changed into fire-love and in this love-fire Christ becomes manifest and is born in the soul. . . . Then from the soul's fire the divine air-spirit proceeds from fire and light and brings its spiritual water out of itself, out of the light. The water becomes essential; and the power of the light eats thereof, and in the love-desire brings itself into a holy being . . . and this being is the true temple . . . yea (it is) God in his own revelation.[25]

Boehme has here explained an authentic mystical experience interpreted through alchemical terminology. It is clearly the same as the devotional use of fire, pneuma *(prāṇa)*, and soma in the generation by reunification of the manifest and unmanifest as Anthropos in the heart during the soma ceremony.

The spiritual water mentioned by Boehme is the same as soma and is the water of life. Speaking of the "water of life," Boehme says, "This water subsists throughout all eternity. It is the water of life which penetrates even death. . . . It is also in the body of man, and when he thirsts for that water and drinks of it, then the light of life is lit in him."[26]

In Boehme's mystical revelation, a subtle pneumatic body of light is formed in the heart, like a pillar of light, which one uses as one's heavenly attire.[27] This is also exactly like the soma tree or pillar of light produced by the entheogenic soma drink. This light form is even more subtle than the star body it projects. The star body is used for miracles and magical operations while still in the physical body. These ideas were derived by Boehme from his readings of Jewish, Latin, and German alchemical texts, along with his own mystical experiences. His sources were ultimately derived from the ancient soma ceremony, but they probably received the information from the later Upaniṣadic sources.

John Dee (1527–1608), magician, mathematician, alchemist, and Kabbalist, used the same sources in constructing his cosmology and in developing his ideas about magic. In Dee's *Monas hieroglyphica* we find seven stages in the cosmological work. He shows the celestial philosophers' egg as containing all creation within it. It is depicted as a downward-pointing egg shape. This suggests the inverted-tree cosmology related to the cosmogonic egg (Fig. 10). He also says that the union of opposites of the higher world of light and dark matter is the source of magic. We have already shown the correspondences between these ideas and the Ṛg Vedic soma ceremony. The most important influences upon Dee's work are revealed in his thoughts on magic and magical practices. As discussed already, earlier Indo-Iranian sacrificial rituals of *haoma*/soma constituted one of the very oldest systemized forms of solar/stellar pneumatic magic ever devised. We can trace its most advanced form back to the Indo-Aryan soma sacrifices of the Ṛg Veda, which had a profound impact upon Neoplatonic magic and theurgy. We also know that Dee's magical thought was mainly influenced by the Islamic philosopher al-Kindī, who, conversely, was mainly influenced by Neoplatonism. Al-Kindī's book on magic, *De radiis*, had a profound effect upon Dee, who is known to have borrowed *De radiis* and to have kept it for two

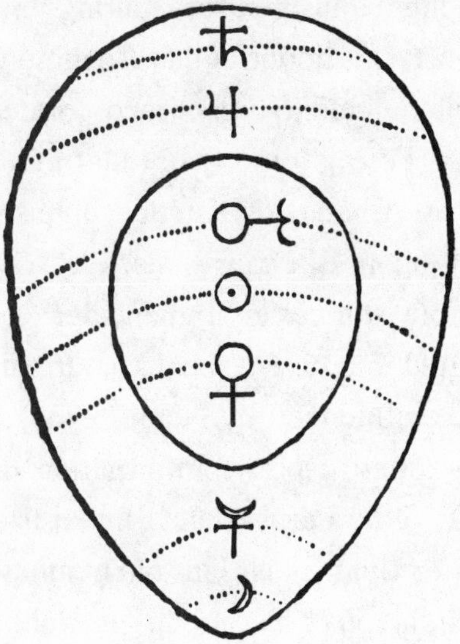

Figure 10. Dee's inverted celestial egg, from his *Monus Hieroglyphica,* Antwerp, 1564.

years. He obviously studied it deeply, as it remains one of the most important sources for Dee's ideas. As Clulee remarks, "The similarity between the wording of passages in al-Kindī and Dee make the dependence of Dee on al-Kindī unquestionable."[28]

Fludd, Boehme, and Dee obtained their symbolism from Jewish mystical works, or directly from Arabic, Hermetic, and Neoplatonic texts whose sources were from India. The doctrines of the Indian Ṛg Veda are thus found in Western kabbalistic, mystical, philosophical, and alchemical treatises, forming an integral part of their practical experiential and cosmological backgound.

Fludd, Boehme, and Dee could have obtained all their information from kabbalistic and alchemical texts, which already contained Indian influences. But a closer source would have been the book *Ein missionsgeschichtlichen Beitragzum Christlichen Dialog mit dem Hinduismus,* written by the Jesuit Robert de Nobili (1577–1656). This book contained a section on the "Theology of the Brahmans." Nobili was a missionary at Madural and Malabar. His book was published and possibly passed around in manuscript form during Boehme, Fludd, and Dee's lifetime. Although it is doubtful that Boehme would have encountered it, it may have been told to him or incorporated into other books he could have read. There is little doubt that this book, plus one other, *China Illustrata* by Athanasius Kircher, published in 1667, had an important impact upon Boehme's disciple, Gichtel. These two books are the probable sources of Indian ideas on the *chakras*, which Gichtel incorporated into his mystical system. Fludd's *chakra* system was probably also influenced by Nobili's book. Both Nobili and Kircher's books contained esoteric information on the *cakra* system based upon the Ṛg Vedic Puruṣa-Sūkta hymn that had been incorporated into various later Upaniṣads. This old hymn is partly the source of the original India *chakra* system. In Nobili and Kircher's works, fourteen centers are located within the primal man as Anthropos, from which the universe is created. Kircher provides an illustration (Fig. 11a) in his book that matches up in many places with Gichtel's chakra system (Fig. 11b), which can be found in his book, *Theosophica practica*, which was published in 1696 although the illustrations were added only in the 1736 edition. Six of Gichtel's seven *chakras* match Kircher's diagram. These are found between the waist and the top of the head. This also accounts for the inaccuracy of the location of the *chakras* in Gichtel's system as compared to authentic Indian texts. Gichtel is thought to have belonged to a secret society of Rosicrucians. He considered this information to be of a secret nature and kept the knowledge hidden for a number of years before publishing it. The subject of his book is mystic regeneration involving the *chakras* and the *elixir vitae* or soma.

a

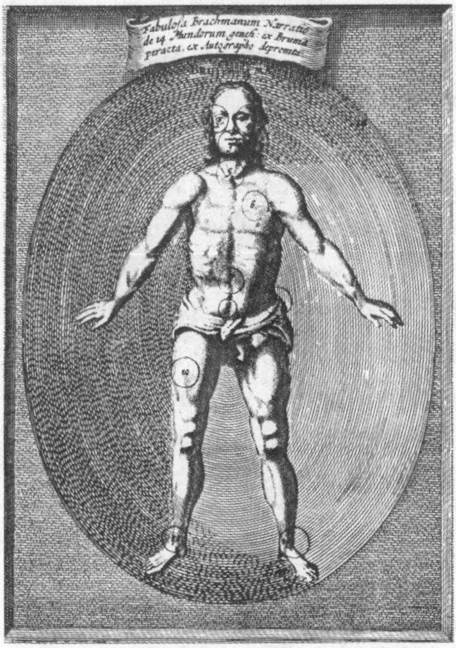

b

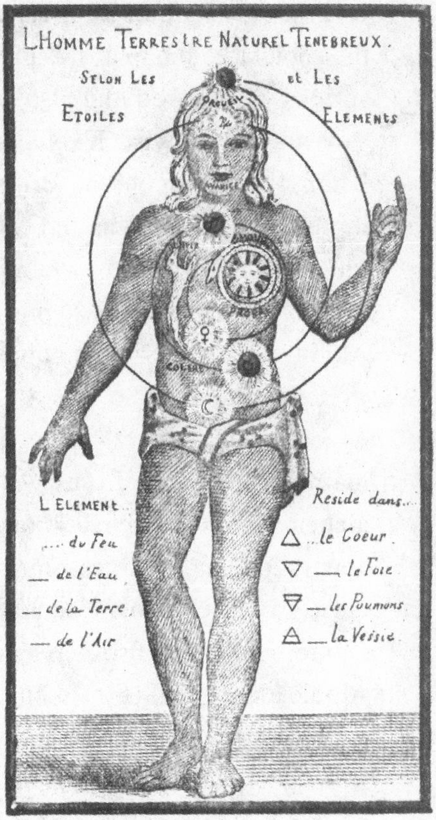

Figure 11. (*a*) Cosmic Anthropos inside the cosmic egg or golden embryo, with Brahmanic *chakra* system from Kircher, *China Illustrata,* 1667; (*b*) Gichtel's *chakra* system, from his *Theosophica practica,* French edition, Paris, 1898.

SOMA, EUROPEAN ELIXIR THEORIES, AND ROGER BACON

In the twelfth century, the translation of Arabic works into European languages began in earnest. There was a medical school at Salerno in southern Italy where translations were prepared and used as early as the eleventh century. The first known translation of an alchemical work from the Arabic was made by Robert of Chester in 1144. By 1200 some half dozen texts had been translated, including the *Book on Alums,* ascribed to al-Razi, and the Emerald Tablet. Interest in the subject began to grow, and in the thirteenth century alchemy was seriously discussed and also widely practiced.

While the Jewish Kabbalists were absorbing Indian ideas from Islam, Roger Bacon, the British scientist, was enthusiastically reading Islamic alchemical and scientific treatises. The best minds of the time doubted whether alchemy was a true science. Saint Albert, also known as Albertus Magnus, Roger Bacon, and Saint Thomas Aquinas all discussed the question of the authenticity of alchemy.[29]

Roger Bacon, who was a practical laboratory worker and a great exponent of the merits of science, discussed the subject of alchemy in many of his books. In his *Opus tertium* he distinguishes speculative alchemy from the actual knowledge of the properties of bodies, their generation, and their transformations. Bacon believed that by the science of alchemy man could perfect metals better and faster than nature could. He also was one of the first Europeans to learn from Arabic alchemical texts about an "elixir of immortality." This ancient elixir appears to have been derived from stories of the soma plant. Regarding alchemy Bacon said, "This science is more important than all that have preceded it because it is productive of more advantage. It not only provides money and infinite other things for the State, but teaches the discovery of such things as how to prolong human life as far as nature allows it to be prolonged."[30] Bacon's science is in many cases what we would call "occult science." He shared the common belief of his time that herbs, stones, metals, and other things possess almost miraculous powers. Bacon often quotes from Artephius concerning the prolongation of life by a secret occult elixir. By thorough investigation of such occult virtues Artephius, exclaims Bacon, prolonged his existence to 1,025 years. Bacon also has unusual occult ideas about the power of the sound of words. He closely connects fascination, the power of words, and the human voice. According to

Bacon, sacred words are the most appropriate instrument, and almost every miracle since the beginning of the world has been performed by using them. Through their power, bodies are healed, venomous animals put to flight, and other such effects produced.[31]

Roger Bacon was convinced that if one conducted a thorough study of nature by direct observation, and studied the ancient philosophers, one would possess great and miraculous secrets. This all sounds naive and humorous to scientists today, but, in fact, Bacon was not so wrong. His only real problem was not having access to competent teachers and better source material in the original languages.

Roger Bacon wanted to be like Artephius, who wisely studied the forces and secrets of nature, especially the secret of the length of life by the development of a miraculous elixir.[32] Bacon's *Mirror of Alchimy* contains, in seven short paragraphs, a manual of alchemical art that teaches how to compose a certain medicine called Elixir, which, when it is projected upon metals or imperfect bodies, makes them perfect at the moment of projection.[33] Bacon had a fascination with the elixir theories he had read about in Arabic sources. In most of his works he mentions longevity and the prolongation of life by these elixirs.

One work translated into English from the Latin was *The Cure of Old Age and the Preservation of Youth*, published in London in 1683. This work quotes many sources, Arabic, Greek, and Chaldean. In this book Bacon writes of a sacred plant of India that bestows longevity and renewed life. He adds that he has obscured and not fully revealed the nature of this plant because it is so powerful that by its use the vulgar might be able to overthrow the entire world and its divine law, and even affect the nature of the universe itself. He says that he is discussing the elixir of life in "obscure and difficult terms which I judge requisite to the conservation of health, least they should fall into the hands of the unfaithful."[34] His descriptions are obscure, but apparently he is describing either one elixir with seven components combined together or seven different elixirs of life, one of them being the "sacred plant of India," which is mentioned as the seventh, and for that reason possibly the most important, elixir. The seven medicines as given by Roger Bacon are, first, that which lies in the bowels of the earth; second, that which lies in the sea; third, that which creeps upon the earth; fourth, that which lives in the air; fifth, that which is like the medicine that comes out of the mineral of the noble animal; sixth, that which comes out of the long-lived animal; and seventh, "that whose mineral is the plant of India."[35] This is of course the inverted mineral stone/plant in previous alchemical texts that we have discussed. It grows in India within the cave of the cosmic mountain, which refers to the structure of the soma ceremony and the soma plant.

Although Bacon does not say what the plant of India is, he does say that it "refreshes the nerves and be-dews them with a thin and subtle moisture, and is good for the brain." He says it "sharpens the senses, cheers the heart."[36] This describes the effects of the "elixir of immortality," the soma drink prepared by the Aśvins. The translator of *The Cure of Old Age*, Richard Browne, writing several hundred years after Bacon, says in his commentary that Roger Bacon is referring to the plant called *Agallochum* or *Lignum Aloes.*[37] Some say it is like a tree with smooth skin rather than bark, that the plant only grows in India, and that there are several types. It is not possible for the translator to have accurately identified this plant from Bacon's work, and he says so. It is not clear what plant Bacon meant; it is clear only that the plant was to be kept secret. Many of the attributes that Bacon gives the plant could also refer to soma. Cosmologically speaking, soma is the prototypical plant of all Indian healing plants and the cosmic tree of the universe.

It is very possible that Bacon could have heard about a sacred plant of India that bestows immortality, longevity, and healing ability and even could transmute lead into gold. He read extensively in Arabic writings on alchemy and the *elixir vitae*. Arabic texts would have certainly referred to the cosmic tree and a sacred plant of India that has the power to heal, rejuvenate, and extend longevity. Bacon, mentioning the mineral of the plant of India, indicates that it may be a mythological plant, and one that is generated through magical means, rather than an actual physical plant. This could mean that he was referring to the subtle essence of the plant, which effects a transformation that directs a person back to the essence of being through the development of the internal pneumatic soma plant.

Bacon was not the only one at this time who was fascinated by the sacred elixir plant of India. Others reading about the marvelous elixir were Arnold of Villanova, who wrote, "Our medicine has also power to heal all infirmity and diseases, both of inflammation and debility; it turns an old man into a youth."[38]

Soma, the Union of Opposites, and the Philosophers' Stone

In European alchemy, the actual preparation of the *elixir vitae* involved the union of opposites within the womb of the heated oven, which is the Hermetic vessel or heart-sun. The symbolism of the union of heaven and earth, sun and moon, and fire and water developed in the soma ceremony was used in alchemical apparatuses such as the altar, throne, and alembic-womb of creation located within the heart of being. The alchemical substances sulphur and mercury were the same as the fire and water or Agni and Soma of the Ṛg Vedic soma ceremony. Once the symbolic union of opposites was achieved, not only were healing and longevity attained, but all sorts of paranormal abilites also resulted.

Mercury and sulphur were not identical with the common substances bearing these names; rather, they stood for cosmic properties inherent in man and the universe, symbolizing the dualistic framework of the cosmos, especially when referred to as "philosophical" mercury or sulphur. Salt was the container that held these two principles; it was known mystically as the body of man and was regarded in alchemical literature as the medium for uniting mercury and sulphur.[39] These three together formed the "triune microcosm," which was the basis of the alchemical cosmology. The union of the two contrary principles (sulphur and mercury) or sun and moon within man's body (salt) forms the immortal pneumatic or astral body used both in the Indo-Aryan soma ceremony and in European alchemy. For example, in the Hermetic alchemical text the Emerald Tablet all the elements found in the Ṛg Veda soma ceremony are present. These elements are the dualistic principles of sun and moon, acted upon by the pneuma to produce the pneumatic fiery golden embryo in the heart. The text says, "Its father is the sun and its mother is the moon. Pneuma is its vital breath . . . these make up the golden embryo."

Allegorical terms such as sulphur, mercury, and salt as well as numerous other symbols were used to veil profound spiritual secrets. These terms continued to increase until the philosophers' stone or elixir was credited with every sort of magical power and paranormal ability known. But we should not discredit these claims, and we should point out that this is exactly what soma stood for and accomplished in the Ṛg Vedic soma ceremony. Some of the soma drinks in the Ṛg Veda, including the *elixir vitae*, were prepared from the alchemical union of dual principles. Sulphur and mercury were frequently mentioned as the sun and moon in European alchemical texts and it was their union or *coniunctionis* that produced the secret "elixir of life." This can be seen in an illustration (Fig. 12) of Hermes pointing to the union of sun and moon, which produces a water that does not burn but gently heats up and illuminates the heart region

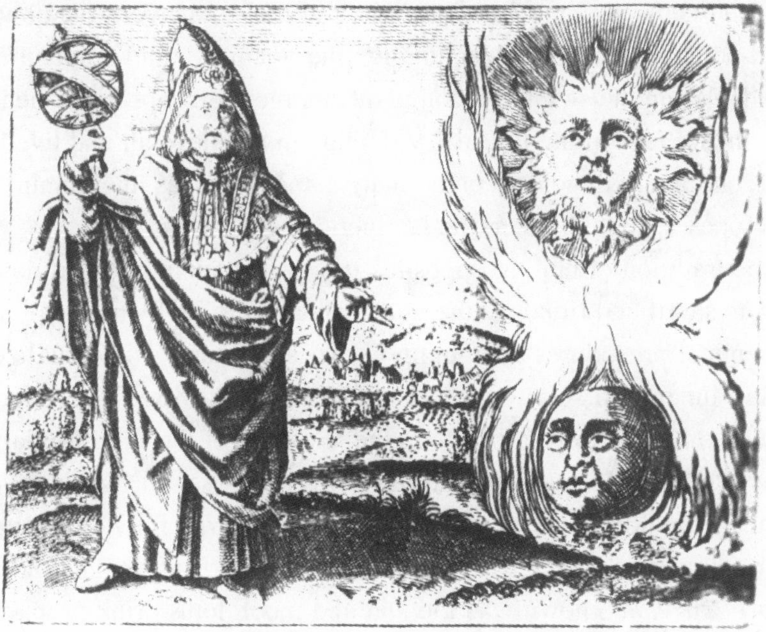

Figure 12. The fiery water that does not burn from the inner union of the sun and moon. From Daniel Stolcius's *Viridarium chymicum*, 1624.

during the inducement of an ecstatic state. This same effect was experienced in the soma ceremony through consuming the entheogenic soma drink.

A direct connection between the preparation of the *elixir vitae* in European alchemy and in the soma ceremony, as the Aśvins' herbal soma drink, can be seen in several European alchemy texts, where the "elixir of life" is said to be prepared directly from the sacred juices of plants that are associated with the symbolic essences of the sun and moon.[40] This is also represented pictorially as sun and moon plants whose sap flows forth through an inverted triangle to produce their equivalents as sulphur 🜍 and mercury ☿ (Fig. 13a). This illustration indicates that the union of the essence or juice of the sun plant, symbolized by sulphur, with the essence or juice of the moon plant, symbolized by mercury, produces the "elixir of life" and inverts the downward-pointing triangle, thus uniting the manifest and unmanifest worlds. When the sun and moon plants merge their saps in the heart, they induce, according to Basil Valentine in his eleventh and twelfth keys, an internal golden plant that is the same as the luminous Anthropos within the heart, the Hermetic vessel[41] (Fig. 13b).

The tradition of uniting opposites is a very ancient one that dates back to sacrificial rituals to the gods, which were really magical and alchemical procedures combining herbal admixtures with ritualized stellar, lunar, and solar operations. These rituals were first systemized by the magi or fire-priests in the fire-cults of the Indo-Iranians. They combined their pneumatic fire rituals with the use of entheogenic drinks, and it was the Indo-Aryans who fully developed their entheogenic drink called soma into the *elixir vitae*. The oldest such *elixir vitae* known was the sun and moon lotus drink prepared by the Aśvins. It was composed of the saps of night-blooming *Nymphaea*, moon plants, mixed with the day-blooming *Nelumbo* and *Nymphaea*, sun plants. Daniel Stolcius in his *Viridarium chymicum,* published in 1624, illustrates the preparation of this *elixir vitae* as the herbal juices of the sun and moon plants, which as John Read mentions, fill the holy grail cup with the "elixir of life" (Fig. 13c). This cup rests upon the sign of both mercury ☿ and gold ☉, symbolizing the golden liquid state of the elixir within the cup of eternity.[42]

There are many different soma drinks and several forms of soma discussed in the Ṛg Veda. The *elixir vitae* that we have mentioned is the golden form of soma consumed as the "elixir of immortality." There is also a white form of soma, which is the celestial soma that is used in the preparation of the *elixir vitae*. This white soma is alchemically changed during the ceremony to golden soma through the ritual heating and mixing process. This white soma is associated with the white stars and the moon. Symbolically it is the same as

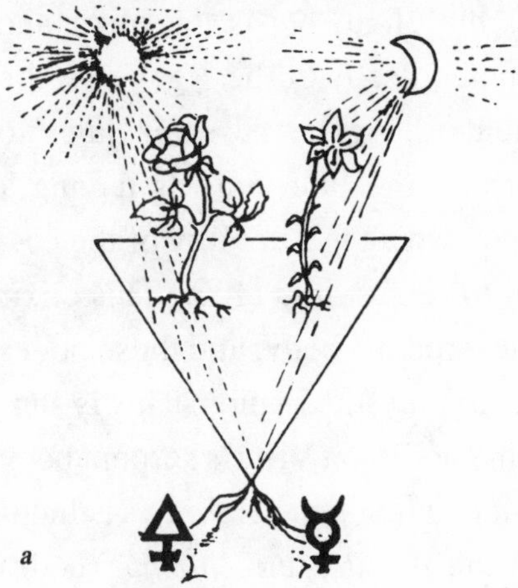

a

b

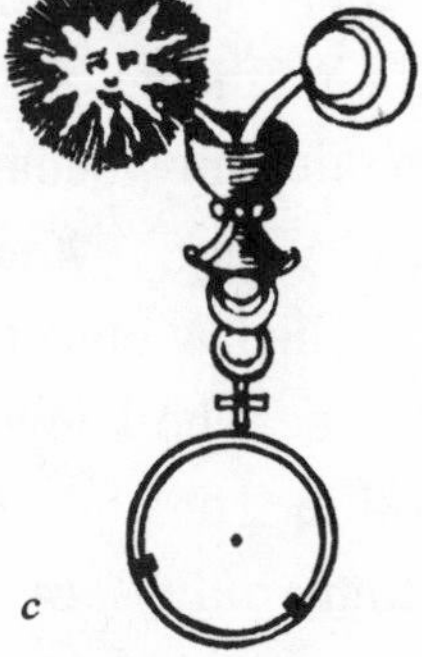

c

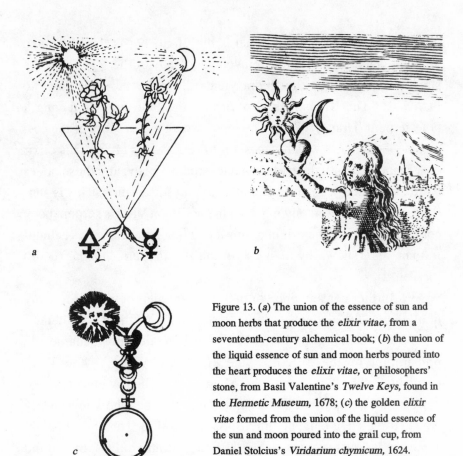

Figure 13. (*a*) The union of the essence of sun and moon herbs that produce the *elixir vitae,* from a seventeenth-century alchemical book; (*b*) the union of the liquid essence of sun and moon herbs poured into the heart produces the *elixir vitae,* or philosophers' stone, from Basil Valentine's *Twelve Keys,* found in the *Hermetic Museum,* 1678; (*c*) the golden *elixir vitae* formed from the union of the liquid essence of the sun and moon poured into the grail cup, from Daniel Stolcius's *Viridarium chymicum,* 1624.

mercury in the European alchemical tradition. The white celestial soma's source, according to the Ṛg Vedic hymns, is the Pole Star. This white soma is also associated with the serpent-dragon Vṛtra in Ṛg Vedic cosmogony. Interestingly, we can find what appears to be an almost direct influence from the Indo-Aryan soma ceremony upon European alchemy in the fact that mercury, also called white water as the "aqua vitae," has its source also at the Pole Star and is associated directly with the serpent-dragon, Draco. Draco is symbolic of immortality and regeneration and guards the white mercurial soma elixir. The serpent not only guards the elixir, but is the elixir and annually sheds its skin and rejuvenates itself. In the Ṛg Veda, the slaying of this dragon by Indra yields this celestial soma juice to mankind.[43] The Kabbalists also viewed the Pole Star as having a pole serpent (Draco), called Teli, upon which the stability of the cosmos depended and which was slain to release the elixir. This elixir was connected with the nodes on the serpent's body, and these nodes were associated with ecstatic states and mystical union. This is similar to the soma ceremony in which the nodes on Vṛtra's serpent body contain the soma. The origin of this idea among the Hebrews is Indo-Iranian, as is shown by their use of the Persian term *juz'har* (node) for Teli.[44]

As a further consequence of their fundamental belief in the unity of all things, the alchemists came to regard the medicine of the metals as the medicine of man. The object of alchemy became the preparation of the "Elixir," "the Heavenly Water," "the Fiery Medicine," "the Phoenix," "the Magistery," which would bring to perfection all imperfect bodies and confer on one who knew rightly how to use them a long, healthy, and vigorous life. The philosophers' stone, under such names as the "Elixir of Immortality" or "Grand Elixir," was depicted as a panacea for all human ills, capable also of restoring youthfulness and prolonging life. The alchemist Ripley made such a claim in the epistle to his *Compound of Alchymie*: "Then will that Medicine heal all manner Infirmities, And turn all Metals to Sun and Moon most perfectly."[45]

In Europe several people had claimed to have actually discovered the philosphers' stone. It is very curious that the stone itself, which we have already shown was also a sacred plant, was still connected directly with India. According to the adept Figuier and others, the alchemists Nicolas Flamel (b. 1330) and his wife Pernelle discovered the philosophers' stone and achieved perennial youth. They were said afterward to have migrated to India; they were said to have lived there as late as the eighteenth century, more than three hundred years after their presumed deaths! It is interesting that they migrated to India, which again indicates that the philosophers' stone had an Indian connection.

Even the longevity of the patriarchs was attributed to their use of the stone. Unless Adam had possessed the knowledge of this great mystery, remarks the author of *Gloria Mundi*, he would not have been able to prolong his life to the age of three hundred, let alone nine hundred, years.

There are even greater wonders. The stone enables one to understand the language of the various creatures, as the chirping of birds, lowing of beasts, and so on. More remarkable still, this stone is not in any way evil or devilish, but easy, natural, and honest.

There is finally the angelical stone, which is so subtle that it cannot be seen, felt, or weighed; it can only be tasted. It enables one to live a long time without food and gives its possessor the power of conversing with angels by dreams and revelations. The alchemist Elias Ashmole (1617–92) has said that Hermes, Moses, and Solomon knew of the secret of this stone, and because of this knowedge they were able to work every kind of wonder.[46]

SOMA AND DESCRIPTIONS OF THE PHILOSOPHERS' STONE

The elixir or philosophers' stone of the alchemist was called by many names that indicate that the real stone, like soma, has an ontological status related to an alteration of one's state of being. These names further show the similarity between the philosophers' stone, or elixir, and soma. The stone was called "Virgin's Milk," "Whiteness,"

"Adam," "Our Great Elixir," "Phoenix," "Universal Medicine," "Yolk of the Egg," "Universal Essence," and the "Water Stone of the Wise" or "Sophic Hydrolith" for its supposed fluid or mercurial appearance.

Zosimos the Panopolitan stated, "In speaking of the Philosopher's Stone, receive this stone which is not a stone, a precious thing which has no value, a thing of many shapes which has not shapes, this unknown which is known of all. . . . The Quintessence is dear and glorious to him who knows it and uses it, vile to him who is ignorant of it; finite and specific for the one, infinite and indeterminate for the other."[47]

The alchemist Eirenaeus Philalethes states in *A Brief Guide to the Celestial Ruby* that "the philosophers' stone is called a stone, not because it is like a stone, but only because, by virtue of its fixed nature, it resists the action of fire as successfully as any stone. In species it is gold, more pure than the purest. If we say that its nature is spiritual, it would be no more than the truth; if we describe it as corporeal, the expression would be equally correct." This type of emphasis was often laid upon the supposed universal occurrence of the stone, and this widespread idea was sometimes advanced as a reason for the cryptic nature of the directions given for its preparation. According to a statement in *Gloria Mundi*, dated 1526,

> The Stone is familiar to all men, both young and old, is found in the country, in the village, in the town, in all things created by God; yet it is despised by all. Rich and poor handle it every day. It is cast into the street by servant maids. Children play with it. Yet no one prizes it, though, next to the human soul, it is the most beautiful and the most precious thing upon earth, and has power to pull down kings and princes. Nevertheless, it is esteemed the vilest and meanest of earthly things.[48]

These statements about the philosophers' stone indicate that it had a spiritual and ontological status just like soma. It was a product of inward operations that created within a person a glorified body possessed of all sorts of miraculous powers. The origins of such ideas, especially once we have seen that the stone was really a plant, come from a probable knowledge of ancient stories about the soma plant and the alchemical processes that derive from the ancient Indo-Aryan soma ceremony.

Alchemy in the Ṛg Veda and the Soma Ceremony

The origin of the idea of the alchemical elixir that can rejuvenate and heal human beings and sustain the entire cosmos as a living entity has its origin in the Indo-Iranian sacrificial ritual of the *haoma*/soma rites. Since these rites are so archaic, they are the probable source of the elixir ideas in Chinese, Greco-Egyptian, Islamic, and European alchemy. In addition, the alchemical concept of spiritual creation and transmutation was also developed within the soma ceremony of the Ṛg Veda.

The earliest forms of rejuvenation in India involve the knowledge of soma, the elixir of life, its source and function in creation, and its activation by fire. These earliest systematized methods of alchemical rejuvenation, using the elixir "soma" or *somarasa* in the rejuvenation of a new body or in the healing of disease, occur primarily in the hymns of the Ṛg Veda and the Atharva Veda. Many of these early methods involve either generating life energy within or pulling life energy into one's body from a macroanthropic process using an entheogenic drink. The rites involve the generation of life energy in the body, bringing it from the source of creation at the cosmic center of the universe, which is centered in man's being at the level of the heart. The soma or elixir is originally located in a place, referred to in the Ṛg Veda as the third heaven, that is situated interdimensionally and microcosmically within the priest's heart/mind. It is also said to be above or beyond the created matter of the stars of the universe. The soma is actually outside the created cosmos, at the cosmic center, within the depths of the watery matrix of creation and being. It is associated with the light energy contained within atoms and the energy that binds together atoms to form molecules of matter. It is associated with the luminous radiant energy of our sun and the stars. It is the foundational energy source from which all other energies and matter are derived. Soma is an energetic luminous fluid that forms a subtle energy body located invisibly inside the physical body, yet extending outside or traveling outside of it. In addition, it is the underlying cause or basis of all physical creation within the creation, as well as that which allows all other space-time dimensions or other worlds to exist. These other worlds are connected to our world by a form of hypercosmic light fluid flowing through the continuum or cosmic pillar.

The entire process of the soma ceremony brings the autonomic processes of the body under conscious control. Small peptide molecules generated within the matrix can pass the blood-brain barrier and be directed to specific sites in the body for healing, rejuvenation, and prolonged life. Some adepts in India suggest that the alchemical elixir or soma of the soma ceremony, when internalized, can be secreted directly from the brain into the bloodstream, keeping the physical body alive even when it is in a state of suspended animation for six months or longer without food, drink, and excretion of waste products. In this state, the body has an extremely low metabolism and a heart rate that is undetectable; there is absolutely no body consciousness and no pain is felt, even if the body is partly eaten by wild animals in the jungle. There is no pain until consciousness is reintroduced into the physical body.

The above example is only one of the many functions of soma and the soma ceremony. It is these types of practices that allow for various control of autonomic processes for healing, rejuvenation, and longevity. It should be noted that gaining control over bodily processes is accomplished not directly through the brain, but through the subconscious mind associated with special states of consciousness. One's essence is approached and identified with again through the true intentions of the heart and spiritual praxis in the heart of being. This process positions one's awareness behind the accumulated impressions of the senses.

The expansion and power of the heart is the greatest force in the universe, and it is fundamental to alchemy. It is a special form of love and is fundamental to our essential nature and consciousness, and it is what controls creation and creative processes. In the soma ceremony the heart is the control point of the forces of nature.

The knowledge of the cosmic tree/pillar as the white *haoma*/soma, and the "elixir of immortality," constitute an ancient system of interior alchemical practice from the oldest books of the Ṛg Veda. If any parts or hymns of the soma ceremony were written before the Indo-Iranians split apart, which appears to be the case, then this knowledge must go back much further. As noted previously, the mythological plant of the Iranian Avesta called the White Hom or *haoma* is the same as the soma of the Ṛg Veda. In the Ṛg Veda the secrets of the soma plant, even though veiled in cryptic language, are fully explained. In the Iranian texts this knowledge about *haoma* is never fully revealed. The Indo-Iranian notion of the cosmic tree/pillar of the universe called the luminous *haoma*/soma is the foundation of their belief system and must be very ancient. Indeed, the date of the *haoma*/soma ceremonies could easily go back to 4000–3000 B.C.E., and current research presents evidence for pushing the date back even further. The Indus culture that appears to have conducted rituals very similar to the soma ceremony has also been shown to be older by the recent discovery of a full-blown writing system already developed by 3500–3300 B.C.E.[49] The Ṛg Veda contains ten books called *maṇḍalas.* From internal evidence and linguistic analysis it can be shown that books two through seven form the oldest core of hymns. Next are books eight and nine. The latest books are one and ten. Some of the information in the books has not been accurately dated. There is internal astronomical evidence in some hymns that some claim date them to around 7000–6500 B.C.E.[50] One important point should be emphasized: Anyone who has read through the thousands of verses of all the books of the Ṛg Veda will quickly realize that they form one cohesive, orderly succession of ideas. The later books, one and ten, only further explain the ideas that are presented in the oldest core books. The later books present not new ideas but simply a representation of the original cosmology as given in the oldest books. Therefore, one is justified in saying that soma, discussed in the core books of the Ṛg Veda, is part of an ancient system of belief.

The ancient soma ritual, as noted, is probably the oldest form of alchemy in the world. The special knowledge of the ritual is used to effect mystical union and healing in the Ṛg Veda, and it formed the foundation of many of the rejuvenative and healing portions of the Atharva Veda. These early systems form the basis of the later alchemical, or *rasāyaṇa,* and Ayurvedic schools of India, as well as other secret healing, longevity, and rejuvenative techniques. Most later techniques of spiritual development in Hinduism, Buddhism, and Jainism are originally derived from parts of the Ṛg Vedic version of the soma ceremony. Both Indian and Tibetan Buddhist schools base their most profound secret inner teachings upon parts of the Ṛg Vedic soma ceremony. Although it is not widely known, Padmasambhava represented a continuation of an ancient miracle tradition associated with the Indo-Iranian magi. In India this tradition derived from the use of the soma drinks and the spiritual basis of the internalized ritual. It is almost certain that Padmasambhava used entheogens in his practices and that he was directly connected with the secret entheogenic use of lotus plants, from which his name (*padma* is Sanskrit for lotus) is derived. The most important teachings of early Tantric and Tibetan Buddhism, as defined in the texts written by Padmasambhava and recently found within the rNying-ma rgyud-'bum, describes the inner generation of the Anthropos of light within the heart. Padmasambhava's full name means "lotus born," which speaks to the birth of the Anthropos from the entheogenic use of the lotus drink. It may also mean the Anthropos is born from the heart as a lotus. Either way, there is little doubt that the internal methods and fundamental ideas of this secret teaching are derived originally from the Ṛg Vedic soma ceremony.[51] The origin of the Tibetan practices of uniting the white and red *bindus* within the heart to form the "ground of being luminosity" comes from the Ṛg Vedic soma ceremony in its uniting of the white celestial soma with the red Agni fire. This practice is basic to most Tibetan Buddhist schools, two of which are the Dzogchen and the Kālacakra.

The soma ceremony of the Ṛg Veda is also the source of ideas about the subtle body in later forms of Indian religion, which connect the subtle body to the *cakra* system of energy centers. Only three such centers are distinguished in the Ṛg Veda soma ceremony. These three centers are the head, heart, and sexual areas, all of which contain vast energy reservoirs. The entheogenic soma ceremony includes methods of dramatically increasing the influx of life energy in these centers, which are brought into alignment to form a luminous pillar and are united in the heart. The later *cakra* system of energy centers along the *suṣumṇā* pillar of light was developed from this original simple system.

The later systems found in various yoga and tantra schools that count four, five, seven, nine, and higher numbers of *chakras* in the subtle body have their origins in the cosmology of the ancient soma ceremony.[52] Even with all the variations and multiplicity of spiritual techniques found in the numerous traditions of India, it is the rather simpler form of the interior soma ceremony by which most saints in ancient and premodern India realized the highest enlightenment. It is also the method they used to work miracles and the basis of the system that is used to heal and extend life.

In all countries in which alchemy has developed we can trace a spiritual as well as a practical or a physical form of development. Although most scholars have concentrated mainly on the physical form, it being the precursor to modern chemistry and metallurgy, the internal spiritual aspects of alchemy, based on ancient sacrificial rites, are older by far than their exterior counterparts. India has had a long history of alchemical practice, as we have shown, but very little work in the West has yet been done toward developing an understanding of its origins, its philosophical framework, and its procedures. As in the European Hermetic tradition, we find in India both a spiritual alchemy connected with the human body and a physical practice using herbs or minerals to restore youth and prolong the life of the body, as well as a combination of the two approaches.

Ṛg Vedic alchemy of the soma ceremony later became intimately connected with the pan-Indian phenomenon of tantra. The origins of alchemy in India have always been associated with the beginnings of tantra. There is, as we have shown, overwhelming evidence of alchemy being practiced in India thousands of years before the advent of the Gupta period (200 B.C.E.–400 C.E.), which is generally acknowledged as the era of the beginnings of tantra, the earliest extant tantric text having been dated no earlier than this period. Even though the texts have been dated to the Gupta period, much of the information they contain is much older. In fact, nearly every idea in later Hindu, Buddhist, and Jain texts that relates to ritual and practice can be traced back to the Ṛg or Atharva Vedas. Although we can determine the approximate date of composition for certain texts, it is very difficult to establish the chronology of philosophical ideas. It is certain that the later forms of Indian yoga, alchemy, and medicine take their forms and practices from the sacrificial rituals of the Vedas, especially the soma sacrifice. In Indian texts, especially the Tantras, it is clearly said that the ideas are simply a revival of forgotten ancient knowledge of the Vedas.[53]

Early Indian alchemy, using soma as the rejuvenative elixir, is primarily concerned with its spiritual side rather than the use of external mineral preparations. In the Ṛg Veda, however, certain plants, among which lotus plants were prominent, were definitely mind altering and used to enhance the internalization of the basic cosmology of the soma ceremony. As noted previously, the soma ceremony itself is of Indo-Iranian origin, and its central idea is of a white or luminous plant that grows from the primal waters of creation to become the living universe. This plant was the white *haoma*/soma; it is an internalized plant that grows from the heart to form the pneumatic body of light.

The ancient soma rituals of the Ṛg Veda provided methods of praxis for internal alchemy and philosophical ideas that were later taken over by both Buddhist and Hindu tantric sects. Alchemy and yoga became covalent within the Indian tantric synthesis. Certain forms of alchemy were simply secret veiled practices of yoga within a tantric framework. Spiritual alchemical practices such as yoga were an internalization of physical ideas based upon the assumption of the correspondence between the microcosm/macrocosm and the union of opposites. Through this internalization, the soma ceremony, alchemy, tantra, and yoga all later became interconnected. This interconnection turned alchemy into another system or means of spiritual perfection with a few new advantages, such as bodily immortality and freedom from all diseases.

It is important to note the difference between immortality and rejuvenation, for it is possible to rejuvenate the body continually for extended periods without reaching immortality, as they are two separate endeavors utilizing some of the same methods. Certainly the soma ceremony of the Ṛg Veda teaches both, but generally, extended longevity leads to immortality. The longevity given by soma is continuous as long as one drinks the soma. The soma ceremony creates a system that allows for perpetual soma production for an eternity. In the Ṛg Veda, the gods who drink soma are given life spans of one thousand years. In the hymns, however, the term *thousand* is figurative and means "infinite," or an "infinite amount of time." This fact is illustrated by the verse in which soma is said to bring wealth "bright with a thousand splendors."[54]

Alchemy, no matter what country it developed in, was always veiled in secrecy. The methods of extraction of the alchemical elixir in the Ṛg Veda are also secret and difficult to understand. Any hymns that refer to the methods always veil the ideas with complicated symbolism that hides their true understanding. The extraction itself is of central importance since *soma* means "to extract" or "press out." This extraction works on multiple levels. The secret, however, lies with the knowledge of the subtle nature of the universe and man, and how this subtle energy is expressed, generated, and identified with during the extraction process. In many cases, the extraction refers to the extraction of the light, both within the microcosm of the physical body and from the celestial soma plant of the third heaven that gives light to the universe. Sometimes the hymns are referring only to the entheogenic soma plant from which the juice is extracted. For a correct reconstruction of the soma ceremony the many levels of the ritual must be understood, which is partly why a clear understanding of the soma sacrifice has remained a mystery for so long.

The internal practices of yoga, particularly those associated with the subtle body, are particularly relevant to alchemy and the soma ceremony. This is true in the Ṛg Veda, but especially so in the later schools of Buddhist Siddhacaryā, among Nātha and Tamil Siddhas, and in the Kālacakra Tantra. The subtle pneumatic body was well known in the Ṛg Veda, and the entheogenic ceremony itself was used to generate it. It was through this body that miracles could be performed. Spiritual elixir alchemy was based upon the consumption of the elixir and the generation of the subtle body. Indian alchemical texts are full of cryptic allusions to the subtle body and its use in alchemical operations. One example is the *Rasārṇavakalpa* (1000 C.E.), which describes the geography of the subtle body, which does not match any earthly sites. The text describes rivers that can only be interpreted as pneumatic and in the subtle body. It speaks of a country called Nagamandala, which confers perfection in all alchemical operations. The rivers it mentions, such as the Sarasvatī, can only be interpreted as pneumatic channels in the subtle body.[55] This example and other Indian alchemical texts indicate that many alchemical operations are conducted through the subtle body. The same is true in European alchemy. Paracelsus says, "Man has an elemental and a super-elemental body—the 'astral body' ('Corpus sidereum'). This is the body which 'teaches man'—for flesh and blood have nothing to impart but carnal desire. Through the astral body man communicates with the super-elemental world of the astra. Its secrets—the 'adepta philosophia' and 'magnalia naturae'—will thus be revealed to him."[56]

Yoga practices, which form the substructure of both Hinduism and Buddhism, have a long history of development in India. Even in the pre-Vedic Indus Valley culture some form of yoga seems to have been practiced. The subtle body, which is so important in alchemy and yoga, has also been understood for a very long time. It was clearly distinguished in the core books of the Ṛg Veda. Knowledge of the subtle body is of particular importance in the soma ceremony, where it is used as the earliest systemized alchemical method of psychogenesis. Knowledge of specific yoga techniques and beliefs concerning the subtle body of light is crucial for an understanding of spiritual alchemy in early Ṛg Vedic India.

The earliest ideas about soma in the Ṛg Veda are closely associated with this subtle body of luminous energy. The "elixir of life" or "water of life" is the radiant energy source that sustains the subtle, interior, immortal body as well as the health of the external, physical body. The seed of this subtle body is the soul or soma itself as the inner sun, the divine spark of God contained in nature that can return to its origin in the realm of the gods. The subtle body is what meditation and the exercises of spiritual alchemy work upon to bring about the healing or rejuvenation of the physical body. This subtle body is intimately connected to consciousness and special states of being, and it is created by means of the logos, pneuma, and entheogens that unify the mind/heart/consciousness complex to devotional one-pointedness.

The early alchemical ideas and practices involving rejuvenation in India depended upon an understanding of man's relationship to the cosmic energies that operate within the universe. These are the energies that create and sustain the entire cosmos, and they are the same energies that man manipulates during the soma ceremony to rejuvenate and organize a new heaven, earth, and solar system. This means that life and the generation or creation of the diversity of species, both plant and animal, are created and maintained on the earth as well as on other worlds in the universe. All of this is done by way of the ancient cosmic ecology of the soma ritual. The term *heaven* here means energy or light, while *earth* means physical matter. There is an important principle in the soma sacrifice that maintains order on earth and in the heavens and brings about the continued formation of new stars and planetary systems within the universe. The soma ceremony maintains the entire universal order of creation, including the physical human body, by using the subtle energies within nature, which were used very early by mankind to alchemically rejuvenate the human body and cure it of disease.

It is in ancient India that specific psychomental healing and rejuvenation techniques were continuously developed, with people being able to heal others and themselves of diseases as well as to increase human life span up to 150 years or longer. In addition, the soma of the Ṛg Veda and Atharva Veda is the source of the alchemical phoenix legends, the Golden Fleece in alchemical tradition and ancient mythology, and "water of life" ideas. The Greek myth of the Golden Fleece has alchemical connotations and is associated with astral gold. In the soma ceremony, a special ritual sieve is prepared specifically from the skin and wool removed from a sacrificial ram. This woolen sieve is used in certain parts of the soma ritual to separate pressed liquid soma from its plant parts. During the movement of the soma liquid to the sieve, other liquids are added before the soma juice reaches the woolen strainer. In the Ṛg Veda, the twin Aśvins are involved in this part of the ritual. As the celestial soma juice passes through it, the white sieve turns a bright golden color. This sieve is made in such a way as to allow seven golden streams to pass through it. The sieve itself becomes symbolic of the birth of the luminous sun and soul as the golden embryo, which contains the elixir of life that flows through it. In European alchemical tradition, ram's wool is said to have been used in sieves for collecting gold from the auriferous rivers of Colchis, which gave rise to the myth of the Golden Fleece. But the myth was also interpreted by alchemists as an allegory of the spiritual journey to discover the "elixir of life." Joseph Pernety interpreted the myth as providing clues to the supreme medicine for the human body.[57] Hermann Fictuld in his *Aureum vellus* (1749 C.E.) says that the "fleece represents the liquid astral gold extracted from the nature of higher realities . . . as a soul and seed, as a solar substance flowing out of God's bounty, it gives life to things, sustains them, and is able to penetrate the most dense and solid bodies." Fictuld says that the elixir is found at the center of some plants.[58] All of what Fictuld says pertains to the Indo-Aryan soma ceremony and the fleece as the sun, which provides the liquid astral gold. This is the same as the solar elixir soma that gives and sustains life. Furthermore, in the Indo-European Greek myth, the twin Dioscuri accompany the Argonauts to seek the Golden Fleece, which represents the sun as a golden embryo. The Dioscuri mirror the twin Aśvins, who at the soma ceremony are involved with the Golden Fleece as the sun and its development into an alchemical golden elixir. Also in the Greek myth, the fleece is hung in a tree, which may symbolize the Ṛg Vedic cosmic tree of the universe. The Golden Fleece itself symbolizes the sun, which sends down its central foot or ray as the central pillar/trunk of the cosmic tree, while its rays are the branches of the tree. The fleece as the sun contains and pours down the golden elixir of life along its branches as sap. In the Greek myth, a dragon guards the Golden Fleece, just as in the Ṛg Veda a dragon called Vṛtra is said to guard the soma.

The soma ritual is also probably one of the oldest systemized uses of an advanced medical/botanical practice using medicinal and hallucinogenic plants and herbs in conjunction with special mental states and rituals. The alchemical elixir that is soma and the internal ecstatic experience created within a person during the soma ceremony paved the way for developments of paranormal pyschogenesis and transmutation in later Hindu, Buddhist, and Jain ascetics. As we can see from many examples, the paranormal activity of transmutation is a special power that is acquired through the internalization of the soma ceremony. The herbal tradition of soma is found in later Buddhist and Hindu sources, where transmutation of any substance into gold can be accomplished through a special state of being induced either by herbal drugs like soma or other means. It is accomplished without any external chemical or electrical means. The *Yoga Sūtras* of Patañjali (300 B.C.E.) say that paranormal powers can be obtained by consuming certain herbs. In the oldest commentary on the sūtras, written by Vyāsa, he says that the herbs refer to the "elixir of life." This connects these herbs directly to the soma drinks in the Ṛg Veda and the paranormal abilities, which are experienced by the *somapas* after drinking soma.[59] In the Avataṃsaka Sūtra (100–300 C.E.), a certain herbal juice or elixir that can change substances into gold is mentioned. The Mahāprajñāpāramitāśāstra of Nāgārjuna, translated into Chinese by Kumārajīva (344–413 C.E.), which is many centuries before Geber (760 C.E.), counts among the *siddhi*, or miraculous powers, the transmutation of stone into gold and gold into stone. Nāgārjuna explains that the transformation of substances can be achieved either by herbs or by the force of the core of being. Furthermore, "by means of herbs and incantations one can change bronze into gold. By a skillful use of herbs, silver may be transformed into gold and gold into silver. By spiritual strength [ecstatic state] man can change clay or stone into gold," says the Mahāprajñāpāramitopadeśa (402 C.E.).[60] Another yoga text says, "One of the siddhis [powers] obtained in yogic practice is 'transmutation of substances into gold.'"[61] Further evidence is given in the following quote, which refers to certain tantric practices within the subtle body.

> He who can gather and hold the red [sun or fire] and white [moon or soma] Tig Les in the Central Channel [*suṣumṇā* as cosmic pillar, will be able to work various kinds of miracles]. . . . He who can bring the Prana-Mind and the pure Essence of the Five Elements into the Central Channel [*suṣumṇā* as cosmic pillar] can:
>
> 1. Transform stones into gold;
> 2. Walk upon water without sinking;
> 3. Enter fire without being burned;
> 4. Travel to a far distant cosmos in a few seconds;
> 5. Fly in the sky and walk through rocks and mountains . . . [62]

The process described here works by uniting the red to the white. But one must know what the red and white really are, and where and how to to unite them. The Ṛg Vedic soma ceremony, more than any other text, tells this secret. In fact, the soma ceremony is the origin of the idea. There are many misunderstandings about how this process is accomplished, even in Buddhist and Hindu texts, since many of these texts were written by scholars who merely compiled the information from other sources without ever having experienced it.

In tantric alchemy, reference is often made to the white and the red, which correlate to soma as mercury and fire as sulphur. These are also referred to as milk and blood as well as semen and ovum. The symbolic terms refer to the two creative and opposing principles in the universe that are brought under control and united by the alchemists. The Hindu Tantra Kāmakalāvilāsa states that the *bindu*, or essence of the universe, consists of two parts: one white, the other red, which represent Śiva as soma and Śakti as fire in the tantric systems. As has been shown, this dualistic symbolism is derived from the union of opposites in the soma ceremony of the Ṛg Veda. Much later they were associated with Śiva and Śakti. Uniting the opposites is considered the method of producing the philosophers' stone. It is also the method of achieving enlightenment in tantric philosophy and the soma ceremony.

This union or coupling together of opposites was symbolized in alchemy as the Hermetic androgyne or hermaphrodite and in the soma ceremony as the rememberment of the primal man of light as Anthropos. This union is frequently represented in tantric statues of Śiva as half male and half female, and it is shown in the soma ceremony as the union of fire and water in the heart and the gathering of soma light essences to reconstitute the primal being of light as the solar heart.

CONCLUSION

There are many correspondences found between the Ṛg Vedic cosmological rituals of the soma ceremony and Chinese, Greco-Egyptian, Islamic, and European alchemy. Not only is soma the probable origin of the elixir ideas in Chinese, Greco-Egyptian, Islamic, and European alchemy, but the cosmological framework of the Ṛg Veda, to which the soma sacrifice is integral, is full of references to what we might call alchemical ideas. The soma ceremony has a basic magical and alchemical cosmology running through it. This is the reason why both Greco-Egyptian and European Hermeticists traced the traditions of magic and alchemy directly back to Indo-Iranian *haoma*/soma sacrificial rituals, which they associated with Zoroaster. Thus in Marsilio Ficino's *Theologia Platonica*, he gives the genealogy of wisdom starting first with Zoroaster, then Hermes Trismegistus, Orpheus, Appollonius, Pythagoras, and finally Plato.[63] As far as the Renaissance Hermetic tradition was concerned, the creation of the "wisdom tradition" and the origins of the "ancient theology" originated with the Indo-Iranians and their *haoma*/soma sacrifices. It was from this tradition that the entheogenic *elixir vitae* was originally conceived.

NOTES

For the sake of simplicity and brevity, these abbreviations have been used in lieu of their corresponding titles throughout the notes that follow:

AV: Atharva Veda

PB: Pañcaviṁśa Brāhmaṇa

RV: Ṛg Veda

SB: Śatapatha Brāhmaṇa

CHAPTER 1

1. The dates of the composition of the Ṛg Vedic hymns continue to be pushed back as more archaeological and textual evidence comes to light. There is archaeological evidence of Indo-Aryans in northern Mesopotamia and Syria before 2000 B.C.E. The Indo-Aryans became eventual rulers of the region. Aryans have been identified with the Kassites of northern Iraq of the eighteenth century B.C.E., and Kassite rulers of Babylon with Indo-Aryan Sanskrit names appear at the beginning of the sixteenth century B.C.E. as do the Mitannian rulers in western Asia in the sixteenth century B.C.E. Ṛg Vedic Sanskrit deities are mentioned in Mitanni treaties around 1450 B.C.E. The Sarasvatī River, mentioned in the Ṛg Veda as a mighty stream, can be used to date many of the hymns before 1500 B.C.E., since the river dried up rapidly after the middle of the second millennium B.C.E.
2. M. Boyce (1989), 1:3.
3. RV 9.44.3; 9.106.4; 9.97.37; 5.44.13, 14, 15. Indra, the main god who drinks soma, becomes stimulated for battle after drinking soma.
4. In RV 10.131, Indra falls down from drinking too much soma.
5. F. E. Peters (1967), p. 57; R. G. Wasson (1979), p. 1.

6. R. G. Wasson (1995), p. 390.

CHAPTER 2

1. RV 4.33; 1.110.4; and F. Neve (1985), pp. 152, 174, fn. 81.
2. J. Sedlar (1980), pp. 208–34.
3. RV 9.113.7.
4. RV 8.79.8; 8.48.4; 8.48.10.
5. Bṛhadāraṇyaka and Chāndogya Upaniṣads, dated 900 B.C.E.
6. It is noteworthy that in a study of 206 subjects who had been given the entheogenic substance LSD, 60% of the subjects reported seeing luminous pillars of light. See R. E. L. and J. Masters (1966), p. 265.
7. R. G. Wasson et al. (1978), p. 37.
8. R. G. Wasson et al. (1978), p. 81.
9. RV 8.14.7.
10. RV 9.110.5; 10.119.8; 8.43.3; 10.31.3.
11. RV 9.113.6.
12. RV 1.165.15; 1.185.9; 7.49.4.
13. RV 8.48.1; 4.26.6.
14. RV 5.40.4; 10.119; 9.113; 8.48; 8.14.7; 1.85.6; 1.85.7.
15. S. Krippner and D. Fersh (1970), pp. 109–14.
16. In the Ṛg and Atharva Vedas, the paranormal effects of soma combined with the ritual of the ceremony are associated with psychogenic creations. RV 3.33; 3.53.9; 7.18.5; 7.33; 2.13.12; 4.19.6; 1.16.11; 1.174.9; 2.15.5; 10.136; 10.119; 10.94.9; 9.73.2; 1.81.5; and 8.88.5.
17. RV 9.90.6; "Long be his life who worships thee [soma]" 9.93.5.
18. RV 9.94.2.
19. RV 9.94.4.
20. RV 4.26.4.
21. RV 9.96.12–14; 4.26.1.
22. RV 9.90.2.
23. RV 9.107.3: "[Soma], the giver of all wealth [immortality], you reside at the cosmic center as a fountain of gold."
24. RV 9.72.6.
25. This cup, out of which the gods drink the elixir of immortality that induces rejuve-

nation and heals the sick, may refer directly to the Grail, which means that the Grail first appears in the oldest Indo-European document, the Ṛg Veda, in association with the soma ceremony.

26. RV 10.97.
27. RV 8.72.17; 8.79.2; 10.25.11; 10.97.18; 8.48.11.
28. RV 1.91.12; 6.74.2–3; 8.20.26; 8.48.5–6, 11; 8.68.2; 9.96.15; 10.76.3; 8.48.6; 8.68.2; 10.25.11.
29. RV 8.48.5, 9; 10.25.11.
30. RV 8.20.26.
31. RV 1.136.6; 6.4.8; 8.48.3, 4, 11; 8.68.6; 9.106.8; 10.144.5, 6.
32. RV 1.126.6; 1.136.6; 6.4.8; 8.83.5; 10.25.8; 10.144.5; 8.91.1; 1.28; 8.31.5.
33. I have completed such a study, and it indicates that the soma drinks did induce interior light phenomena, and that this special experience was a fundamental part of soma inebriation, in addition to being the interior microcosmic cosmography of the ceremony itself. Depending on the strength of the compounds and what plants were used to prepare soma, it could have effects that include photic visionary experiences, as well as consciousness-enhancing and calming effects that could allow ecstatic states to manifest during the ritual. A state of deep calm and well-being, which is fundamental for ecstasy, also sharpens mental faculties so that word associations flow naturally for poetically inspired compositions, which is another characteristic of soma inebriation, since many of the hymns in the Ṛg Veda appear to have been composed after drinking soma.

CHAPTER 3

1. For extensive documentation of the identity of both the *haoma* and soma plants, as well as a reconstruction of the Ṛg Vedic soma ceremony and its underlying cosmology, see my forthcoming *Soma: Plant of Immortality.*
2. D. Chakrabarti (1990).
3. Both *Nymphaea* and *Nelumbo* plants worldwide are little understood and have not been studied pharmacologically in any comprehensive way. Many misconceptions currently exist about the relationship between the two genera as well as the alkaloids and other compounds that are found in both. I have studied the folklore and medicinal and pharmacological aspects of both genera, and I have researched the psychoactive and medicinal effects found in various naturally occurring wild *Nelumbo*, *Nymphaea*, and *Nuphar* species described in a number of languages, including Sanskrit, Chinese, Japanese, French, German, English, Greek, Hindi, Arabic, Spanish, and Polish. See Spess and Reding (2000).

4. RV 1.135.4; 3.40.1; 5.34.2.
5. RV 9.1.4; 9.86.44.
6. Direct references to *Nelumbo* or *Nymphaea* species occur in the Ṛg Veda eight times, but indirect references to these plants are much more numerous.
7. Besides the lotus only a few other flowers are directly mentioned, such as the flowers of the *simbal* and *śālmali* trees.
8. RV 8.4.12.

CHAPTER 4

1. RV 8.22.8.
2. RV 10.184.3; AV 3.22.4.
3. RV 10.106.6.
4. Mahābhārata, 1.66.40.
5. RV 8.10.1.
6. RV 1.46.2–6.
7. RV 1.119.9; 1.112.21; SB 4.1.5.17; 14.5.5.16.
8. RV 1.180.1–2; 1.182.2; 1.183.4; 3.58.4; 10.40.6; 10.41.3; 1.34.10.
9. RV 10.61.15; 8.82; 8.26.6.
10. RV 1.112.21.
11. RV 4.45.4.
12. RV 9.26.1.
13. RV 5.75.6; 1.181.2.
14. RV 1.47.8.
15. RV10.75.8
16. RV 10.97.7.
17. RV 1.116.7.
18. RV 1.180; 1.181; 1.182; 1.183; 1.184.
19. AV 6.69.1; 9.1.18–19.
20. PB 14.11.26.
21. RV 1.191.10.
22. SB 5.1.2.10.
23. RV 2.41.14; 9.77.1 VS 21.
24. RV 8.8.4; 7.67.4.
25. RV 1.34.3.

26. RV 1.157.6.
27. RV 10.106.6–7; 1.157.4; 8.68.5–6; 1.20.3; 10.39.12; 10.5.6 describes travel to other worlds along the branches of the cosmic tree of light.
28. RV 8.9.20; 10.106.11; 1.112.20; 8.9.21.
29. RV 4.45.4.
30. RV 1.157.6.
31. RV 8.22.15–16; 4.45.4.
32. L. Farnell (1970), p. 210.
33. RV 8.48.
34. RV 1.117.22.
35. RV 8.5.6.
36. RV 8.8.3–5; 4.14.4.

CHAPTER 5

1. J. W. McCrindle (1881), pp. 18, 25, 31, 34, 61.
2. Budge (1899).
3. B. Puri (1939), p. 40.
4. J. W. McCrindle (1881), pp. 47–48.
5. J. W. McCrindle (1960), pp. 76–79; on soma as a type of wine, see Rawlinson (1926), p. 58.
6. J. Sedlar (1980).
7. Rooke (1813), p. 219.
8. J. Edkins (1900), p. 590.
9. J. Needham (1974), vol. 5, part 2, pp. 115, 121–22; (1980), vol. 5, part 4, p. 504.
10. S. K. Lakshminarayana (1970), p. 26.
11. H. Yule (1920), vol. 2, pp. 365–66.
12. G. Boas (1948), pp. 160, 161.
13. E. W. Hopkins (1905), p. 12.
14. M. Z. Siddiqi (1959), pp. 30, 33, quotes from "Amr b. Bahr al-Jahiz of Basra (d. 869 C.E.) and from the Arabic book '*Arab wa Hind ke Ta'alluqat,* pp. 3, 12, 71–72.
15. Serpents were known to rejuvenate themselves by shedding their skin. In the Ṛg Veda soma is also compared to a serpent that sheds its skin and rejuvenates itself.
16. J. Needham (1974), vol. 5, part 2, pp. 492–98; see also J. Needham (1981).
17. V. Karmarkar (1950), p. 25.

18. H. P. Yoke (1982), p. 35.
19. L. Kohn (1993), p. 4.
20. O. S. Johnson (1928), pp. 47–50; K. J. DeWoskin (1983), pp. 18, 140–53, 188n.127.
21. The classic explication of immortality as the goal of breath control is found in H. Maspero (1981), pp. 459–554; see also N. Sivin (1968), pp. 31–32.
22. J. Needham (1983), vol. 5, part 5, p. 280.
23. J. Filliozat (1949), pp. 113–120.
24. M. Eliade (1958), p. 59; J. Needham (1983), vol. 5, part 5, p. 288.
25. RV 4.42.3.
26. L. Wieger (1969), pp. 395–97, 401, 403, 405.
27. W. E. Soothill (1925), pp. 16, 18; L. Wieger (1969), p. 367.
28. J. Filliozat (1969), p. 46.
29. L. Gwei-Djen (1973), p. 72.
30. J. Needham (1980), vol. 5, part 4, pp. 292–300, discusses the egg, womb, and elixir embryo.
31. Ibid., p. 245.
32. Ibid., p. 244.
33. W. Bauer (1976), pp. 91, 104, 159, 165, 390.
34. H. H. Dubs (1947), p. 62; J. Needham (1974), vol. 5, part 2, p. 115.
35. J. Needham (1974), vol. 5, part 2, p. 117.
36. Ibid.
37. Ibid., p. 118.
38. Ibid., p. 121.
39. A. Waley (1930), pp. 22–23.
40. A. Waley (1932), p. 1102; J. Needham (1983), vol. 5, part 5, pp.22–23: "Waley then pointed out how in later times Taoist *nei tan* alchemy was much influenced by Buddhism, especially of the Chhan or Zen School, as the case of Ko Chhang-Keng, also known as Pai Yu Chhan, whose *Hsiu Hsien Pien Huo Lun* (Resolution of Doubts Concerning the Restoration to Immortality) written about +1218, shows explicitly. Thus Waley touched the very essence of the matter by demonstrating that alchemical terminology had been transferred from a specifically chemical-metallurgical context to a psycho-physiological one, *nei tan* 'elixirs' and their components not being in crucibles or retorts but in the actual organs and vessels of the human body."
41. J. Lindsay (1970), p. 93.

42. Ibid., pp. 97–101.
43. Ibid., p. 101.
44. R. Multhauf (1966), pp. 83–84, 114.
45. F. Cumont (1912), p. 58.
46. J. Lindsay (1970), p. 150.
47. Ibid., p. 345.
48. M. Z. Siddiqi (1959), pp. 32–33.
49. Ibid., p. 33–34.
50. Ibid., p. 34.
51. Ibid., pp. 34–35.
52. D. M. Bose (1971), p. 318, quoting from Ramadevar's *Cunnakandam*, 227, 466.
53. H. P. Yoke (1982), p. 35.
54. I. Shah (1964), pp. 194, 196.
55. H. E. Stapleton (1927), pp. 389–411.
56. H. E. Stapleton (1953), p. 17, n. 30, 38. This is an important point because dualist theories make up the basis of both alchemical theory as well as the Indo-Aryan soma sacrifice, which indicates that Indo-Iranian cosmological ideas underlie the very foundations of alchemy.
57. F. S. Taylor (1949), pp. 78–79.
58. S. H. Nasr (1968), p. 31.
59. Quoted in R. V. Patvardhan (1920), vol. 1, p. clv.
60. S. H. Nasr (1978), p. 247.

CHAPTER 6

1. J. V. Prasek (1906), vol. 1, p. 62.
2. B. Hrozny (n.d.), p. 182.
3. W. F. Albright (1940), p. 31; R. Drews (1988), p. 227.
4. I. Puskas (1987), p. 147.
5. F. Graf (1997), p. 20.
6. C. H. Kahn (1979), pp. 262, 297–302; M. L. West (1971), pp. 111–202.
7. F. Graf (1997), pp. 27–28.
8. M. L. West (1971), pp. 206–8.
9. Ibid., pp. 62–68.
10. P. Kingsley (1995), pp. 233–49.

11. H. Lambridis (1976), pp. 12–13; M. R. Wright (1981), pp. 11–14.
12. F. Graf (1997), p. 33.
13. P. Kingsley (1995), pp. 223, 226–27; H. Lambridis (1976), pp. 120–21.
14. Diogenes Laertius (1925), 8.2.6.
15. Philostratus (1912); G. Anderson (1986).
16. F. Petrie (1908), p. 129.
17. M. Murray (1961), p. 318.
18. See all of the evidence given by Z. P. Thundy (1993), pp. 174–252.
19. R. T. Wallis (1972), pp. 47–72.
20. There is some hint of this view in Assyrian texts, but only in an embryonic form, which had already been greatly influenced by Indo-Aryan religion of the Mitanni centuries before.
21. Porphyry (1969), part 10.
22. A. Riginos (1976), pp. 66–67, 165–66.
23. R. T. Wallis (1972), pp. 14, 15.
24. See R. B. Harris (1982).
25. R. T. Wallis (1972) p. 35.
26. Ibid., p. 108–9.
27. J. F. Finamore (1985), pp. 167–69.
28. G. Luck (1985), pp. 22–23.
29. G. Shaw (1995), pp. 221–28.
30. H. Lewy (1978), pp. 399–441; R. B. Harris (1982), pp. 1–345; J. F. Staal (1961), pp. 1–249; R. T. Wallis (1972), p. 15, n.2.
31. R. T. Wallis (1972) p. 86.
32. Z. P. Thundy (1993); J. Sedlar (1980), pp. 199–208.
33. E. Conze (1970), pp. 651–67; R. Garbe (1959), pp. 70–123; J. Sedlar (1980), pp. 107–252. See also G. Filoramo (1990), pp. 44, 129; K. Rudolph (1983), pp. 60, 86, 132.
34. See G. Filoramo (1990), pp. 112–13; K. Rudolph (1983), pp. 75–76, 95ff, 337.
35. For a full summary of different scholars' views and their conclusion that the Anthropos is of Iranian origin, see C. H. Kraeling (1927).
36. R. C. Zaehner (1955), p. 137: "There seems to be every reason to believe that this is a case of Indian influence on Iranian thought." See also W. N. Brown (1931 and 1942).

37. C. H. Kraeling (1927), p. 190.
38. M. L. West (1971), pp. 87–98, 105–8.
39. C. H. Kraeling (1927), pp. 109–10.
40. H. Jonas (1958), pp. 216–37.
41. Van Nooten (1994), p. 455; RV 9.74.2.
42. RV 10.90.2ab.
43. RV 6.9.6, trans W. Johnson (1982), p. 57.
44. A. De Conick (1996), pp. 64–85.
45. Ibid., pp. 157–72.
46. R. Reitzenstein (1978), pp. 426–500.
47. J. D. Tabor (1986); B. A. Pearson (1973); M. Smith (1973), pp. 220–48; G. Wagner (1967), pp. 9–11.
48. S. Gunduz (1994), p. 86.
49. H.-J. Klimkeit (1982), p. 11.
50. H. Jonas (1958), p. 60.
51. G. Widengren (1963), pp. 205–17. C. H. Dodd showed that both the Christian ideas of baptism and the Anthropos, derived from soma, were from Indo-Iranian sources via Mandaean schools. There is also a similar influence upon the ideas found in the Fourth Gospel. See Casey (1964), p. 54.
52. On magical practices and ascension in relation to the Merkabah, see I. Gruenwald (1980).
53. G. Scholem (1965).
54. N. Deutsch (1995), pp. 68–79.
55. J. Elias (1995), p. 81; M. J. Winston (1981), pp. 161–63.
56. On Indian influences in the development of the Imam concept, see M. A. Amir-Moezzi (1994), pp. 94–95, 181. On the Imam connected to the cosmic pillar, Pole Star, and sun, see H. Corbin (1978).
57. D. L. Gelpi (1984), pp. 116–18.
58. H. Jackson (1978).
59. G. R. S. Mead (1919), p. 28.
60. M. Boyce (1989), p. 24, n. 9; L. Woolley (1953), p. 82–83.
61. B. P. Copenhaver (1992), pp. 3–4, 106–10.
62. C. H. Kraeling (1927), p. 76.
63. C. H. Dodd (1953), pp. 264–65.

64. K. W. Luckert (1991), pp. 135–39.
65. B. Shafer (1991), pp. 95–96
66. See also E. L. Miller (1989).
67. K. Rudolph (1983), pp. 77, 85, 131, 143, 144, 149, 305; G. Filoramo (1990), pp. 11, 26, 76, 107, 79, 213, 41, 42, 62, 113, 66, 76, 117, 160.
68. G. R. S. Mead (1919), pp. 60, 66.
69. P. Kristeller (1964), p. 371.
70. Plato obviously obtained his conceptions of the star body found in his *Phaedrus* and *Timaeus* from Indian sources who knew of the Ṛg Veda. The way Plato's ideas are mixed up, they appear to be a combination of Babylonian astrology and Indian cosmology. It can be shown that Plato was influenced by Indo-Iranian religions and that the theory of both the immortal subtle starlike body as well as the so-called mortal astral body were derived from the theological background of the soma ceremonies. These subtle forms are not originally derived from either Plato or Aristotle, as E. R. Dodds tried to show ([1963], pp. 313–21).
71. G. Widengren (1963), pp. 205–17.
72. F. Lamplugh (1918), pp. 14–15; V. MacDermot (1978), pp. 242, 247, 227; C. A. Baynes (1933), pp. 3–190.

CHAPTER 7

1. S. Parpola (1993), p. 191.
2. In a treaty excavated at Bogaz Koy, between the kingdoms of Mitanni and Egypt, that can be dated to around 1400 B.C.E., the Sanskrit names of Indo-Aryan gods are mentioned. Mitra is a deity used to seal contracts and treaties. Yet the mention of Varuṇa, Mitra, Indra, and the twin Aśvins together possibly had an important meaning because of the combined role they performed in the Mitanni ritual.
3. S. Parpola (1993), p. 191.
4. M. Lurker (1980), pp. 70–71.
5. D. T. Potts (1992). For a detailed study see D. L. Spess (2000).
6. A. Daniélou (1973), p. 139.
7. F. M. Cornford (1952), p. 353.
8. A. Kaplan (1982), pp. 156, 330.
9. G. Scholem (1965), pp. 104, 112–15, 128; S. Fisdel (1996), pp. 177–83.
10. "Now the Tree of Life extends from above downward" *Zohar* (n.d), vol. 5, p. 203; *Bahir* (1979), pp. 34, 38, 45, 67; G. Scholem (1987), p. 76, further explains the concept of the inverted tree in the *Bahir.*

11. G. Scholem (1987), pp. 78–80.
12. G. Nigal (1994), pp. 51–66.
13. *Bahir* (1979), p. 38, sec. 102; G. Scholem (1987), p. 154.
14. R. C. Zaehner (1961), pp. 20–21; M. Haug (n.d.), pp. 4, 30, 31, 192, 216, 301, 303, 311; G. Carter (1918), pp. 1–106.
15. M. Idel (1988), pp. 14, 24, 25, 39; G. Scholem (1961), pp. 139–55.
16. C. G. Jung (1983), pp. 460, 410.
17. This text is taken from the book *The Secrets of Alchemy*, composed by Galid, the son of Jazich, translated from Hebrew into Arabic and from Arabic into Latin and from Latin into English. This work is contained within Roger Bacon's *The Mirror of Alchimy* (1597). Our version is an adaptation from S. J. Linden (1992), p. 41; and R. Patai (1994), pp. 130–31.
18. C. G. Jung (1983), p. 410; quotes from Ventura, *De ratione conficiendi lapidis, in theatrium chemicum* (1659), vol. 2, p. 226 and *Musaeum Hermeticum*, pp. 240, 270.
19. C. G. Jung (1983), p. 422; quote from Johann Daniel Mylius, *Philosophia reformata* (1622), p. 260.
20. C. G. Jung (1983), p. 423; quotes from *Ars Chemica*, p. 160; H. Khunrath, *Von hylealischen . . . Chaos*, p. 20.
21. C. G. Jung (1983), pp. 380–81; quote from *Theatricum Chemicum* (1659), vol. 1, p. 513.
22. W. Huffman (1988), p. 60.
23. R. Fludd (1982), p. 15.
24. J. Boehme (1794).
25. J. Boehme (1930), pp. 152–53.
26. M. Aniane (1953), p. 65.
27. H. Martensen (1949), p. 178.
28. N. Clulee (1988), p. 255 n. 45.
29. F. S. Taylor (1949), pp. 94–95.
30. Ibid., pp. 97–98. Roger Bacon, *Opera quaedam bactenus inedita*, ed. J. S. Brewer (1859) pp. 39–40. The subject is also discussed in most of Bacon's other works.
31. L. Thorndike (1923), pp. 664–66.
32. T. L. Davis (1923), p. 35.
33. E. Westacott (1955), p. 66.
34. R. Bacon (1683), p. 15.
35. Ibid., p. 16.

36. Ibid., pp. 87–88.
37. Ibid., p. 92.
38. Quoted in J. Read (1937), p. 123.
39. Ibid., pp. 25, 27, 28.
40. J. D. Mylius (1622), p. 313.
41. B. Valentine (1893), vol. 2, p. 348.
42. J. Read (1937), pp. 104–5.
43. Ibid., pp. 100, 105; C. G. Jung (1976), p. 484; C. G. Jung (1977), p. 188.
44. A. Kaplan (1990), pp. 232–37.
45. J. Read (1937), p. 123.
46. Ibid., pp. 125–26.
47. Ibid., p. 129.
48. Ibid., pp. 129–30.
49. M. Kenoyer (1999), p. 15.
50. S. Kak (1994); G. Feuerstein et al. (1995), p. 107. Both of these books give evidence from internal astronomical information contained within the hymns of the Ṛg Veda that date those books to 6500 B.C.E. or earlier.
51. On the Anthropos and the formation of a subtle anthropocosmic body of light generated in the heart as the basic teachings of Padmasambhava and the foundation of his methods of producing miracles, see Guenther (1996), pp. 8, 53, 56, 63, 65, 68, 105, 106 n. 91, 169. On soma as the elixir of immortality located in the heart of being, see p. 158. Because the inner Anthropos of light within the heart is part of Padmasambhava's mystical teachings, Guenther suspected that Padma had come into contact with Western Gnostic ideas concerning the Anthropos. This would be a reasonable assumption if one did not know or understand the teachings contained within the Ṛg Vedic soma ceremony, teachings that are much older than Gnosticism, and whence the Gnostic schools derived the idea of the Anthropos.
52. Four centers are found in most tantric Buddhist schools (see Dasgupta [1974]); five are found in the Hindu tantric Kubjikamatatantra; seven are found in most Hindu tantric systems; and nine are found in some Kashmiri Hindu systems.
53. A. Wayman (1982).
54. RV 9.12.9.
55. *Rasārṇavakalpa*, verses 628–94.
56. W. Pagel (1958), p. 120.
57. A. Faivre (1990), pp. 251–53.

58. A. Faivre (1993), p. 41.

59. Patañjali: 4.1, 6; M. R. Yardi (1979), pp. 236, 238.

60. M. Eliade (1962), p. 131.

61. From the Yogatattva Upaniṣad, translated in Aiyar (1980), p. 197.

62. C. C. Chang (1963), pp. 79–80.

63. C. Butler (1970), p. 50; D. Horst (1964), pp. 268–69.

BIBLIOGRAPHY

Aiyar, K. Narayanasvami. (1980). *Thirty Minor Upanishads: Including the Yoga Upanishads.* With an introduction by David Spess. Boulder: Santarasa Publications.

Albright, William F. (1940). "New Light on the History of Western Asia in the Second Millennium B.C." *Bulletin of the American Schools of Oriental Research.* 77–78; 20–32; 23–31.

Ameisenowa, Z. (1938). "The Tree of Life in Jewish Iconography." *Journal of the Warburg Institute* 2:326–45.

Amir-Moezzi, Mohammad Ali. (1994). *The Divine Guide in Early Shi'ism: The Sources of Esotericism in Islam.* Albany: State University of New York Press.

Anderson, Graham. (1986). *Philostratus.* London: Croom Helm.

Aniane, Maurice. (1953). "Notes sur l'alchimie, yoga cosmologique de la chretiente medievale." Translated into English as "Notes on Alchemy the Cosmological Yoga of Medieval Christianity" in *Material for Thought* (Spring 1976): 55–96.

Apte, Vaman Shivaram. (1986). *The Practical Sanskrit-English Dictionary.* Revised and enlarged edition. Kyoto: Rinsen Book Company.

Apte, Vaman Shivaram. (1993). *The Student's English-Sanskrit Dictionary.* Delhi: Motilal Banarsidass.

Arapura, J. G. (1975). "The Upside Down Tree of the Bhagavad Gita." *Numen* 22: 131–44.

Atharva Veda. (1909). *The Parisistas of the Atharvaveda.* Vol. 1, pt.1. Edited by George

Melville Bolling and Julius von Negelein. Leipzig: Otto Harrassowitz.

Atharva Veda. (1960–1962). *Atharvaveda (Saunaka) with the Pada-patha and Sayanacarya's Commentary.* Edited by Vishva Bandhu, et al. 4 vols. Hosiapur: Vishveshvaranand Vedic Research Institute.

Atharva Veda. (1966). *Atharva-Veda-Saṃhitā.* Edited by Herausgegevan von R. Roth and W. D. Whitney. Bonn: Ferd. Dummlers.

Atharva Veda. (1979). *Atharvaveda of the Paippaladas.* Edited by Raghu Vira. Sasasvati Vihara Series 1, 9, 12. Delhi: Arsh Sahitya Prashar Trust.

Atharva Veda. *Les Hymnes Rohitas. L'Atharva-Veda,* vol. 13. Trans. and ed. Victor Henry. Paris: J. Maisonneuve.

Atharva-Parisista. Edited by Ram Kumar. Varanasi: Chaukhambha Orientalia, 1976.

Bacon, Roger. (1683). *The Cure of Old Age and the Preservation of Youth.* London: Tho. Flesher.

Bahir. (1979). Translated into English from the Hebrew by Aryeh Kaplan. New York: Samuel Weiser.

Barret, LeRoy Carr. (1993). "Three Versions of an Atharvan Hymn." In *Oriental Studies in Honour of Cursetiji Erachji Pavry.* Ed. Jal Dastur Cursetiji Pavry. London: Oxford University Press.

Bauer, Wolfgang. (1976). *China and the Search for Happiness.* New York: Seabury Press.

Baynes, C. A. (1933). *A Coptic Gnostic Treatise Contained in the Codex Brucianus.* Cambridge: Cambridge University Press.

Beal, Samuel. (1964). *Travels of Fah-hian and Sung-yun, Buddhist Pilgrims, From China to India (400 A.D. and 518 A.D.).* London: Susil Gupta.

Bhawe, S. S. (1957–62). *The Soma-Hymns of the Ṛgveda: A Fresh Interpretation.* 3 vols. Baroda: Oriental Institute.

Bidez, J., and F. Cumont. (1973). *Les Mages Hellenises: Zoroastre Ostanes et Hystaspe d'Apres la Tradition Grecque.* 2 vols. Paris: Societe d'Edition Les Belles Lettres.

Boas, George. (1948). *Primitivism and Related Ideas in the Middle Ages.* Baltimore: Johns Hopkins Univ. Press.

Boehme, Jacob. (1794). *The Works of Jacob Boehme.* 4 vols. London: G. Robinson.

Boehme, Jacob. (1930). *The Election of Grace.* Trans. by John Rolleston Earle. London: Constable.

Bolle, Kees W. (Ed.). (1987). *Secrecy in Religion.* Leiden: E. J. Brill.

Bose, D. M. (1971). *A Concise History of Science in India.* New Delhi: The Indian National Science Academy.

Boyce, Mary. (1989). *A History of Zoroastrianism.* Vol. 1. Leiden: E. J. Brill.

Brown, W. Norman. (1931). "The Sources and Nature of Puruṣa in the Puruṣasūkta (Rigveda 10.91). *Journal of the American Oriental Society* 51:108–118.

Brown, W. Norman. (1942). "The Creation Myth of the Rig Veda." *Journal of the American Oriental Society* 62:85–98.

Budge, Wallis. (Trans.). (1899). *The History of Alexander the Great Being the Syriac Version.* Cambridge: Cambridge University Press.

Budge, Wallis. (1904). *The Book of Paradise.* Vols. 1 and 2. New York: G. P. Putnam's Sons.

Burns, J. Edgar. (1969). *The Art and Thought of John.* New York: Harper and Row.

Burrows, T. (1973). *The Sanskrit Language.* London: Faber and Faber.

Butler, Christopher. (1970). *Number Symbolism.* London: Routledge & Kegan Paul.

Carter, George. (1918). *Zoroastrianism and Judaism.* Boston: The Gorham Press.

Casey, R. P. (1964). "Gnosis, Gnosticism and the New Testament." In *The Background of the New Testament and Its Eschatology.* Ed. by W. D. Davies and D. Daube. Cambridge: Cambridge University Press.

Chakrabarti, Dilip K. (1990). *The External Trade of the Indus Civilization.* New Delhi: Munshiram Manoharlal.

Chang, C. C. (1963). *Teachings of Tibetan Yoga.* New York: University Books.

Clulee, Nicholas. (1988). *John Dee's Natural Philosophy.* New York: Routledge.

Conze, Edward. (1970). "Buddhism and Gnosis." In *Le Origini dello Gnosticismo.* Leiden: E. J. Brill.

Coomaraswamy, A. K. (1938). "The Inverted Tree." *Quarterly Journal of the Mythic Society* (Bangalore) 29:111–49.

———. (1970). "Khawaj Khadir and the Fountain of Life, in the Tradition of Persian and Mughal Art." *Studies in Comparative Religion* 4 (4): 221–30.

Copenhaver, Brian P. (1992). *Hermetica: The Greek* Corpus Hermeticum *and the Latin* Asclepius *in a New English Translation, with Notes and Introduction.* Cambridge: Cambridge University Press.

Corbin, Henry. (1978). *The Man of Light in Iranian Sufism.* Boulder: Shambala.

Cornford, Francis Macdonald. (1952). *Plato's Cosmology: The Timaeus of Plato, Translated with a Running Commentary.* London: Routledge & Kegan Paul.

Cumont, Franz. (1912). *Astrology and Religion Among the Greeks and Romans.* London: Constable.

Daniélou, Alain. (1973). *Yoga: The Method of Re-Intergration.* London: Johnson

Publications.

Dasgupta, S. B. (1974). *An Introduction to Tantric Buddhism.* Calcutta: University of Calcutta.

Davis, Tenney L. (1923). *Roger Bacon's Letter: Concerning the Marvelous Power of Art and of Nature and Concerning the Nullity of Magic.* Easton, Penn.: Chemical Publishing Co.

De Conick, April. (1996). *Seek to See Him: Ascent and Vision, Mysticism in the Gospel of Thomas.* Leiden: E. J. Brill.

Deutsch, Nathaniel. (1995). *The Gnostic Imagination: Gnosticism, Mandaeism, and Merkabah Mysticism.* Leiden: E. J. Brill.

DeWoskin, Kenneth J. (Trans.). (1983). *Doctors, Diviners, and Magicians of Ancient China: Biographies of Fang-shin.* New York: Columbia University Press.

Diogenes Laertius. (1925). Trans. from the Greek by R. D. Hicks. Vols. 1 and 2. Cambridge: Harvard University Press.

Dodd, C. H. (1953). *The Interpretation of the Fourth Gospel.* Cambridge: Cambridge University Press.

Dodds, E. R. (1963). *Proclus, the Elements of Theology: A Revised Text with Translation, Introduction and Commentary.* Second ed. Oxford: Oxford University Press.

Doniger, Wendy. "Somatic Memories of R. Gordon Wasson." In *The Sacred Mushroom: Seeker Essays for R. Gordon Wasson.* Ethnomycological Studies, no. 11. Foreword by Richard Schultes. Historical, Ethno- & Economic Botany Series. Vol. 4. Portland: Dioscorides Press.

Drews, Robert. (1988). *The Coming of the Greeks, Indo-European Conquests in the Aegean and the Near East.* Princeton: Princeton University Press.

Drower, E.S. (1960). *The Secret Adam: A Study of Nasoraean Gnosis.* Oxford: Oxford University Press.

Dubs, H. H. (1947). "The Beginnings of Alchemy." *Isis* 38 (62).

Dumont, P. E. (1939). *L'Agnihotra: Description de l'agnihotra dans le rituel vedique d'apres les Srautasūtras.* Baltimore: Johns Hopkins University Press.

Edkins, Joseph. (1900). *China Review.* Williams, reprint of 1900 edition. Smithsonian Institute. xiii, 411, 590.

Ehrich, Robert W. (Ed.). (1992). *Chronologies in ancient world Archaeology.* 2 vols. Chicago: University of Chicago Press.

Eliade, Mircea. (1958). *Yoga: Immortality and Freedom.* Bollingen Series 56. Princeton: Princeton University Press.

Eliade, Mircea. (1962). *The Forge and the Crucible.* New York: Harper & Brothers.

Eliade, Mircea. (1964). *Shamanism: Archaic Techniques of Ecstasy.* Bollingen Series 86. Princeton: Princeton University Press.

Eliade, Mircea. (1965). *Mephistopheles and the Androgyne: Studies in Religious Myth and Symbol.* New York: Sheed & Ward.

Elias, Jamal. (1995). *The Throne Carrier of God: The Life and Thought of Ala Ad-dawala As-Simnani.* Albany: State University of New York Press.

Faivre, Antoine. (1989). "An Approach to the Theme of the Golden Fleece in Alchemy." In Z. R. W. M. von Martels. Alchemy Revisited: Proceedings of the International Conference on the History of Alchemy at the University of Groningen 17–19 April 1989. Leiden: E. J. Brill. 250–58.

Faivre, Antoine. (1993). *The Golden Fleece and Alchemy.* Albany: State University of New York Press.

Faivre, Antoine. (1995). *The Eternal Hermes.* Grand Rapids, Mich.: Phanes Press.

Faraone, C. A., and Dirk Obbink. (1991). *Magika Hiera: Ancient Greek Magic and Religion.* New York: Oxford University Press.

Farnell, Lewis Richard. (1970). *Greek Hero Cults and Ideas of Immortality.* Oxford: Oxford University Press.

Feuerstein, Georg et al. (1995). In Search of the Cradle of Civilization: New Light on Ancient India. Wheaton, Ill.: Quest Books.

Filliozat, Jean. (1949). "Taoisme et Yoga." *Dan Viet Nam* 3:113–20.

———. (1969). "Taoisme et Yoga." *Journal Asiatique* 257:41–87.

Filoramo, Giovanni. (1990). *A History of Gnosticism.* Oxford: Basil Blackwell.

Finamore, John F. (1985). *Iamblichus and the Theory of the Vehicle of the Soul.* Chico, Calif.: Scholars Press.

Fisdel, Steven. (1996). *The Practice of Kabbalah: Meditation in Judaism.* Northvale: Jason Aronson, Inc.

Fludd, Robert. (1982). *Utriusque Cosmi Historia.* Translated into English by Patricia Tahil as the Origin and Structure of the Cosmos of Books One and Two of Tractate One from Volume One. Edinburgh: Magnum Opus Hermetic Sourceworks.

Gangopadhyaya, M. (1981). *Indian Atomism: History and Sources.* Atlantic Highlands: Humanities Press.

Garbe, Richard. (1959). *India and Christendom: The Historical Connections between Their Religions.* La Salle, Ill.: Open Court.

Gelpi, Donald L. (1984). *The Divine Mother: A Trinitarian Theology of the Holy Spirit.* Lanham: University Press of America.

Gichtel, J. G. (1898). *Theosophia Practica.* Paris: Bibliotheque Chacornac.

Graf, Fritz. (1997). *Magic in the Ancient World.* Cambridge: Harvard University Press.

Gruenwald, Ithamar. (1980). *Apocalyptic and Merkabah Mysticism.* Leiden: E. J. Brill.

Guenther, Herbert. (1996). *The Teachings of Padmasambhava.* Leiden: E. J. Brill.

Gunduz, Sinasi. (1994). *The Knowledge of Life, The Origins and Early History of the Mandaeans and Their Religion to the Sabians of the Qur'an and to the Harranians.* London: Oxford University Press.

Gwei-Djen, Lu. (1973). "The Inner Elixir (Nei Tan): Chinese Physiological Alchemy." In Teich, Mikulas, and Robert Young. *Changing Perspectives in the History of Science: Essays in Honour of Joseph Needham.* Boston: D. Reidel Publishing Company.

Harris, R. Baine. (Ed.). (1982). *Neoplatonism and Indian Thought.* Albany: State University of New York Press.

Haug, Martin. (n.d.). *Essays on Sacred Language, Writings, and Religion of the Parsis.* London: Kegan Paul, Trench, Trubner & Company.

Hirst, Desiree. (1964). *Hidden Riches.* London: Eyre & Spottiswoode.

Hopkins, Edward W. (1905). *The Religions of India.* Boston: Ginn & Company.

Hrozny, Bedrich. (n.d.). *Ancient History of Western Asia, India and Crete.* Prague: Artia.

Huffman, William. (1988). *Robert Fludd and the End of the Renaissance.* London: Routledge.

Hume, Robert E. (1921). *The Thirteen Principal Upanishads, Translated From the Sanskrit.* London: Oxford University Press.

Idel, Moshe. (1988). *The Mystical Experience in Abraham Abulafia.* Albany: State University Press of New York.

Jackson, Howard. (Ed. and trans.). (1978). *Zosimos of Panopolis on the Letter Omega.* Missoula: Scholars Press.

Jackson, Williams. (1932). *Researches in Manichaeism.* New York: Columbia University Press.

Johnson, Obed S. (1928). *A Study of Chinese Alchemy.* Shanghai: The Commercial Press, Ltd.

Johnson, Willard. (1982). *Riding the Ox Home: A History of Meditation from Shamanism to Science.* London: Rider & Company.

Jonas, Hans. (1958). *The Gnostic Religion: The Message of the Alien God and the Beginnings of Christianity.* Boston: Beacon Press.

Jung, C. G. (1976). *Mysterium Coniunctionis.* Vol. 14, *Collected Works.* Princeton: Princeton University Press.

Jung, C. G. (1977). *Psychology and Alchemy.* Vol. 12, *Collected Works.* Princeton: Princeton University Press.

Jung, C. G. (1983). *Alchemical Studies.* Vol. 13, *Collected Works.* Princeton: Princeton University Press.

Kahn, Charles H. (1979). *The Art and Thought of Heraclitus.* Cambridge: Cambridge University Press.

Kak, Subhash. (1994). *The Astronomical Code of the Ṛg Veda.* New Delhi: Aditya.

Kaplan, Aryeh. (1982). *Meditation and Kabbalah.* York Beach, Maine: Samuel Weiser.

Kaplan, Aryeh. (1990). *Sefer Yetzirah.* York Beach, Maine: Samuel Weiser.

Karmarkar, V. (1950). *Religions of India: The Vrātya or Dravidian Systems.* Lonavala.

Kashmirian Atharva Veda. (1936). "The Kashmirian Atharva Veda, Books 16 and 17." Edited by LeRoy Varr Barret. New Haven: *Journal of the American Oriental Society* 9.

Kashmirian Atharva Veda. (1940). "The Kashmirian Atharva Veda, Books 19 and 20." Edited by LeRoy Carr Barret. New Haven: *Journal of the American Oriental Society* 18.

Kashmirian Atharva Veda. (n.d.). "The Kashmirian Atharva Veda, Book 6." Edited by Franklin Edgerton. *Journal of the American Oriental Society* 34:374–411.

Kashmirian Atharva Veda. (n.d.). "The Kashmirian Atharva Veda, Books 1–5, 7–15, 18". Edited by LeRoy Carr Barret. *Journal of the American Oriental Society* 26:197–295; 30:187–258; 32:343–90; 35:42–101; 37:257–308; 40:145–69; 41:264–89; 42:105–46; 43:96–115; 44:258–69; 46:34–48; 47:238–49; 48:34–65; 50:43–73; 58:571–614.

Kenoyer, Mark. (1999). "Early Indus Script." *Archaeology.* Sept./Oct. 1999:15.

Kingsley, Peter. (1995). *Ancient Philosophy, Mystery and Magic: Empedocles and Pythagorean Tradition.* Oxford: Oxford University Press.

Kippenberg, Hans G., and Guy G. Stroumsa. (Eds.). (1995). *Secrecy and Concealment: Studies in the History of Mediterranean and the Near Eastern Religions.* Leiden: E. J. Brill.

Klimkeit, Hans-Joachim. (1982). *Manichaen Art and Calligraphy.* Leiden: E. J. Brill.

Kohn, Livia. (1993). *The Taoist Experience: An Anthology.* Albany: State University of New York Press.

Kraeling, Carl H. (1927). *Anthropos and Son of Man: A Study in the Religious Syncretism of the Hellenistic Orient.* New York: Columbia University Press.

Krippner, Stanley, and Don Fersh. (1970). "Paranormal Experience Among Members of American Contra-Cultural Groups." *Journal of Psychedelic Drugs* 3 (1):109–14.

Kristeller, Paul. (1964). *The Philosophy of Marsilio Ficino.* Gloucester: Peter Smith.

Lakshminarayana, S. K. (1970). *A History of Medicine, Surgery and Alchemy in India.* Tenali: Published by the author.

Lambridis, Helle. (1976). *Empedocles: A Philosophical Investigation.* Alabama: The

University of Alabama Press.

Lamplugh, F. (1918). *The Gnosis of the Light: A Translation of the Untitled Apocalypse Contained in the Codex Brucianus.* London: John M. Watkins.

LaPlante, Eve. (1993). *Seized, Temporal Lobe Epilepsy as a Medical, Historical, and Artistic Phenomenon.* New York: HarperCollins.

Lewy, Hans. (1978). *Chaldaean Oracles and Theurgy.* Paris: Etudes Augustiniennes.

Linden, Stanton J. (Ed.). (1992). *The Mirror of Alchimy, Composed of the Thrice-Famous and Learned Friar, Roger Bachon.* New York: Garland Publishing.

Lindsay, Jack. (1970). *The Origins of Alchemy in Graeco-Roman Egypt.* London: Frederick Muller.

Lowe, J. E. (1929). *Magic in Greek and Latin Literature.* Oxford: Basil Blackwell.

Luck, Georg. (1985). *Arcana Mundi: Magic and the Occult in the Greek and Roman Worlds.* Baltimore: John Hopkins University Press.

Luckert, Karl W. (1991). *Egyptian Light and Hebrew Fire.* Albany: State University of New York Press.

Lurker, Manfred. (1980). *The Gods and Symbols of Ancient Egypt.* London: Thames and Hudson.

MacDermot, Violet. (1978). *The Books of Jeu and the Untitled Text in the Bruce Codex.* Leiden: E. J. Brill.

MacDonnell, A. A. (1991). *A Practical Sanskrit Dictionary with Transliteration, Accentuation, and Etymological Analysis Throughout.* New York: Oxford University Press.

Mallory, J. P. (1989). *In Search of the Indo-Europeans. Language, Archaeology and Myth.* London: Thames and Hudson.

Martensen, Hans. (1949). *Jacob Boehme: Studies in His Life and Teaching.* London: Rockliff.

Maspero, Henri. (1981). *Taoism and Chinese Religion.* Amherst: The University of Massachusetts Press.

Masters, R. E. L., and Jean Masters. (1966). *The Varieties of Psychedelic Experience.* London: Anthony Blond. Reprint (2000). Rochester, Vt.: Park Street Press.

McCrindle, J. W. (Trans.). (1881). "Ancient India as Described by Ktesias the Knidian." *Indian Antiquary* 18.

McCrindle, J. W. (Trans.). (1960). *Ancient India as Described by Megasthenes and Arrian; Being a Translation of the Fragments of the Indika of Megasthenes Collected by Dr. Schwanbeck, and of the First Part of the Indika of Arrian.* Rev. 2nd ed. Calcutta: Chuckervertty, Chatterjee & Co.

Mead, G. R. S. (1919). *The Doctrine of the Subtle Body in Western Tradition.* London: Stuart & Watkins.

Miller, Ed L. (1989). *Salvation-History in the Prologue of John: The Significance of John 1: 3/4.* Leiden: E. J. Brill.

Monier-Williams. (1979). *A Sanskrit-English Dictionary.* Oxford: Oxford University Press.

Multhauf, Robert. (1966). *The Origins of Chemistry.* London: Oldbourne.

Murray, Margaret. (1961). *The Splendor That Was Egypt.* New York: Philosophical Library.

Mylius, Johann Daniel. (1622). *Philosophia Reformata.* Frankfurt: Lucas Jennis.

Nasr, Seyyed Hossein. (1968). *Science and Civilization in Islam.* Cambridge: Harvard University Press.

Nasr, Seyyed Hossein. (1978). *An Introduction to Islamic Cosmological Doctrines.* London: Thames & Hudson.

Needham, Joseph. (1974). *Science and Civilization in China.* Vol. 5, part 2. Cambridge: Cambridge University Press.

Needham, Joseph. (1980). *Science and Civilization in China.* Vol. 5, part 4. Cambridge: Cambridge University Press.

Needham, Joseph. (1981). *Science in Traditional China.* Cambridge: Harvard University Press.

Needham, Joseph. (1983). *Science and Civilization in China.* Vol. 5, part 5. Cambridge: Cambridge University Press.

Needham, Joseph. (1986). *Science and Civilization in China.* Vol. 6, part 1. Cambridge: Cambridge University Press.

Neve, Felix. (1985). *An Essay on the Myth of the Ṛbhus.* Translated from the French by G. V. Davane. Delhi: Ajanta Publications.

Nigal, Gedalyah. (1994). *Magic, Mysticism, and Hasidism: The Supernatural in Jewish Thought.* Northvale: Jason Aronson, Inc.

O'Flaherty, Wendy Doniger. (1968). "The Post-Vedic History of the Soma Plant." In *Soma: The Divine Mushroom of Immortality.* Ed. R. Gordon Wasson. Ethno-mycological Studies, no. 1. The Hague: Mouton and Co.

O'Flaherty, Wendy Doniger. (1986). *The Ṛg Veda.* New York: Penguin.

Otto, Walter F. (1965). *Dionysus Myth and Cult.* Bloomington: Indiana University Press.

Pagel, Walter. (1958). *Paracelsus.* New York: S. Karger.

Pancavimsa Brāhmaṇa. (1931). Translated into English by W. Caland. Calcutta: Asiatic Society.

Parpola, Simo. (1993). "The Assyrian Tree of Life: Tracing the Origins of Jewish Monotheism and Greek Philosophy." *Journal of Near Eastern Studies* 52(3):161–208.

Patai, Raphael. (1994). *The Jewish Alchemists: A History and Source Book.* Princeton: Princeton University Press.

Patvardhan, R. V. (1920). "Rasavidyā or Alchemy in Ancient India." In *Proceedings and Transactions of the First Oriental Conference.* Vol. 1. Poona: Bhandarkar Oriental Research Institute.

Pearson, Birger Albert. (1973). *The Pneumatikos-Psychikos Terminology in 1 Corinthians; A Study in the Theology of Corinthian Opponents of Paul and its Relation to Gnosticism.* Missoula: Scholars Press.

Peters, F. E. (1967). *Greek Philosopical Terms: A Historical Lexicon.* New York: New York University Press.

Petrie, Sir Flinders. (1908). *Man.* Vol. 8.

Philostratus. (1912). *The Life of Apollonius of Tyana.* 2 vols. Loeb Classical Library. Trans. F. C. Conybeare. Cambridge: Harvard University Press.

Pliny. (1962). *Selections from the History of the World Commonly Called the Natural History of C. Plinius Secundus.* Translated into English by Philemon Holland, Doctor in Physics, and Selected and introduced by Paul Turner. London: Centaur Press.

Porphyry. (1969). *Ad Marcellam.* Edited with German translation and commentary by W. Potscher. Leiden: E. J. Brill.

Potts, D. T. (1992). *The Arabian Gulf in Antiquity.* Vol. 1. Oxford: Oxford University Press.

Prasek, J. V. (1906). *Geschichte der Meder und Perser bis sur Makedonischen Eroberung.* 2 vols. Gotha: Germany.

Puri, Baij. (1939). *India as Described by Early Greek Writers.* Lucknow: Indological Book House.

Puskas, Ildiko. (1987). "Trade Contacts Between India and the Roman Empire." 141–56. In Pollet, Gilbert. (Ed.). *India and the Ancient World History, Trade and Culture Before A.D. 650.* Leuven: Dept. Orientallistiek.

Rasārṇavakalpa. (ca. 1100 C.E.). Photocopy of manuscript in Nagara script from the University of Delhi.

Rawlinson, H. G. (1926). *Intercourse between India and the Western World from the Earliest Times to the Fall of Rome.* 2nd edition. Cambridge: Cambridge University Press.

Read, J. (1937). *Prelude to Chemistry: An Outline of Alchemy, Its Literature and Relationships.* New York: Macmillian.

Reitzenstein, Richard. (1978). *Hellenistic Mystery-Religions: Their Basic Ideas and Significance.* Translated from the German by John Steely. Pittsburgh: The Pickwick Press.

Ṛg Veda. (1951–1957). *Der Rig-Veda, aus dem Sanskrit ins Deutsche Ubersetzt.* Edited by Karl Friedrich Geldner. 4 vols. Harvard Oriental Series 33–36. Cambridge: Harvard University Press.

Ṛg Veda. (1966). *The Hymns of the Rig-Veda with Sayana's Commentary.* 4 vols. Edited by F. Max Muller. The Chowkhamba Sanskrit Series 99. Varanasi: The Chowkhamba Sanskrit Series Office.

Ṛg Veda. (1977). *Ṛgveda-Sarvanukramani of Katyayana and Anuvakanukramani of Saunaka.* Edited by Umesh Chandra Sharma. Aligarh: Viveka Publications.

Ṛg Veda (1994). *Rig Veda: A Metrically Restored Text with an Introduction and Notes.* Edited by B. Van Nooten and Gary Holland. Cambridge: Harvard University Press.

Riedlinger, Thomas. (1990). *The Sacred Mushroom Seeker: Essays for R. Gordon Wasson.* Ethnomycological Studies, no. 11. Foreword by Richard Schultes. Historical, Ethno- & Economic Botany Series. Vol. 4. Portland: Dioscorides Press. Reprint (1997). Rochester, Vt.: Park Street Press.

Riginos, A. (1976). *Platonica: The Anecdotes Concerning the Life and Writings of Plato.* Leiden: E. J. Brill.

Rooke, M. (1813). *The Expedition of Alexander the Great, and Conquest of Persia.* Translated from the original Greek. Second ed. London: J. Davis.

Rudolph, Kurt. (1983). *Gnosis: The Nature and History of Gnosticism.* New York: Harper & Row.

Sarup, Lakshman. (1967). *The Nighantu and the Nirukta, The Oldest India Treatise on Etymology, Philology, and Semantics.* Delhi: Motilal Banarsidass.

Śatapatha-Brāhmaṇa. (1897). *The Śatapatha-Brāhmaṇa According to the Text of the Madhyandina School.* Translated by Julius Eggeling. 5 vols. Oxford: The Clarendon Press.

Scholem, Gershom. (1961). *Major Trends in Jewish Mysticism.* New York: Schocken Books.

Scholem, Gershom. (1965a). *Jewish Gnosticism, Merkabah Mysticism, and Talmudic Tradition.* New York: Jewish Theological Seminary.

Scholem, Gershom. (1965b). *On the Kabbalah and its Symbolism.* New York: Schocken Books.

Scholem, Gershom. (1987). *Origins of the Kabbalah.* Princeton: Princeton University Press.

Sedlar, Jean. (1980). *India and the Greek World.* Totowa, N. J.: Rowman and Littlefield.

Sen, S. N. (1963). "Transmission of Scientific Ideas Between India and Foreign Countries in Ancient and Medieval Times." *Bulletin of the National Institute of Sciences of India* 21:8–30.

Sen, S. N. (1966). "An Estimate of Indian Science in Ancient and Medieval Times." *Scientia:* 123–134.

Shafer, Byron. (Ed.). (1991). *Religion in Ancient Egypt. Gods, Myths, and Personal Practice.* Ithaca: Cornell University Press.

Shah, Idries. (1964). *The Sufis.* New York: Doubleday.

Shaw, Gregory. (1995). *Theurgy and the Soul: The Neoplatonism of Iamblichus.* University Park: University of Pennsylvania Press.

Siddiqi, Muhammad Zubayr. (1959). *Studies In Arabic And Persian Medical Literature.* Calcutta: Calcutta University.

Sivin, Nathan. (1968). *Chinese Alchemy: Preliminary Studies.* Cambridge: Harvard University Press.

Smith, Morton. (1973). *Clement of Alexandria and a Secret Gospel of Mark.* Cambridge: Harvard University Press.

Soothill, W. E. (1925). *China and the West: A Sketch of Their Intercourse.* London: Oxford University Press.

Spess, David L. (2000). *Soma, Plant of Immortality: A Comprehensive Study Including a Reconstruction of the Ṛg Vedic Soma Ceremony.* Taos: Codex Press.

Spess, David L., and Katherine E. Reding. (2000). *Flowers of Ecstasy and Immortality: The Folklore, Medicinal Uses, and Psychopharmacology of Sacred Lotus and Water Lily Plants of Egypt and India.* Taos: Codex Press.

Staal, J. F. (1961). *Advaita and Neoplatonism: A Critical Study in Comparative Philosophy.* Madras: University of Madras.

Stapleton, H. E. (1927). "Chemistry in Iraq and Persia in the Tenth Century A.D." *Memoirs of the Asiatic Society of Bengal* 8(6):317–418. Calcutta: The Asiatic Society of Bengal.

Stapleton, H. E. (1953). "The Antiquity of Alchemy." *Ambix: The Journal of the Society for the Study of Alchemy and Early Chemistry* 5 (1 and 2):1–43.

Stroumsa, Guy. (1996) *Hidden Wisdom: Esoteric Tradition and the Roots of Christian Mysticism.* Leiden: E. J. Brill.

Tabor, James D. (1986). *Things Unutterable: Paul's Ascent to Paradise in its Greco-Roman, Judaic and Early Christian Contexts.* Lanham: University Press of America.

Taylor, F. Sherwood. (1949). *The Alchemists: Founders of Modern Chemistry.* New York: Henry Schuman.

Thorndike, Lynn. (1923). *A History of Magic and Experimental Science.* Vol. 2. *During the First Thirteen Centuries of Our Era*. New York: Columbia University Press.

Thorwald, Jurgen. (1963). *Science and Secrets of Early Medicine*. New York: Harcourt, Brace, and World.

Thundy, Zacharias P. (1993). *Buddha and Christ: Nativity Stories and Indian Traditions*. Leiden: E. J. Brill.

Vaitana. Saṃhitā. (1974). Edited by Vishva Bandhu. Hoshiarpur: V.V.R.I.

Valentine, Basil. (1893). *The Twelve Keys of Basilius Valentinus the Benedictine*. In *The Hermetic Museum*. 2 vols. London: Elliot Stock. Vol. 1, pp. 324–57.

Wagner, Gunter. (1967). *Pauline Baptism and the Pagan Mysteries: The Problem of the Pauline Doctrine of Baptism in Romans VI. I–II, in the Light of Its Religio-Historical "Parallels."* Edinburgh: Oliver and Boyd.

Waley, Arthur. (1930). "Notes on Chinese Alchemy." *Bulletin of the School of Oriental Studies London Institution* 6(1):1–24.

Waley, Arthur. (1932). "References to Alchemy in Buddhist Scriptures." *Bulletin of the School of Oriental Studies* 6(4):1102–3.

Wallis, R. T. (1972). *Neoplatonism*. New York: Charles Scribners & Sons.

Wasson, R. Gordon. (1968). *Soma: The Divine Mushroom of Immortality*. Ethno-mycological Studies, no. 1. The Hague: Mouton and Co.

Wasson, R. Gordon. (1971). "The Soma of the Ṛg Veda: What was it?" In Ernest Bender (ed.), *R. Gordon Wasson on Soma and Daniel H. H. Ingalls' Response*. American Oriental Series, no.7. New Haven: American Oriental Society.

Wasson, R. Gordon. (1972). "Soma and Fly-Agaric." *Ethhno-Mycological Studies* 2. Botanical Museum of Harvard University.

Wasson, R. Gordon. (1979a) "Foreword to a Book Catalogue." *Phantastica: Rare and Important Psychoactive Drug Literature, 1700 to the Present*. Introduction by Michael Horowitz. Los Angeles: Pegacycle.

Wasson, R. Gordon. (1979b). "Soma Brought Up-To-Date." *Journal of the American Oriental Society* 99(1):100–105.

Wasson, R. Gordon. (1980). *The Wondrous Mushroom: Mycolatry in Mesoamerica*. New York: McGraw Hill.

Wasson, R. Gordon. (1995). "Ethnomycology: Discoveries About *Amanita muscaria* Point to Fresh Perspectives." In *Ethnobotany: Evolution of a Discipline*. Ed. Richard Evans Schultes. Portland: Dioscorides Press.

Wasson, R. Gordon et al. (1978). *The Road to Eleusis: Unveiling the Secret of the Mysteries*. New York: Harcourt Brace Jovanovich.

Wasson, R. Gordon et al. (1986). *Persephone's Quest: Entheogens and The Origins of Religion*. New Haven: Yale University Press.

Wayman, Alex. (1982). "The Human Body As Microcosm in India, Greek Cosmology, and Sixteenth-Century Europe." *History of Religions* 22(2):172–90.

West, M. L. (1971). *Early Greek Philosophy and the Orient.* Oxford: Oxford University Press.

Westacott, E. (1955). *Roger Bacon: In Life and Legend.* London: Rockliff.

Widengren, Geo. (1963). "Baptism and Enthronement in Some Jewish-Christian Gnostic Documents." In S. G. F. Brandon. *The Saviour God: Comparative Studies in the Concept of Salvation Presented to Edwin Oliver James.* Manchester: Manchester University Press. pp. 205–217.

Wieger, Leo. (1969). A *History of the Religious Beliefs and Philosophical Opinions in China From the Beginning to the Present Time.* New York: Paragon Book Reprint

Wilson, William J. (1940). "The Background of Chinese Alchemy." *Ciba Symposia:* 594.

Winston, Morris James. (1981). *The Wisdom of the Throne: An Introduction to the Philosophy of Mulla Sadra.* Princeton: Princeton University Press.

Wirgin, Wolf. (1964). "The Menorah as Symbol of After-Life." *Israel Exploration Journal* 4:102–104.

Wohlberg, Joseph. (1990). "Haoma-Soma in the World of Ancient Greece." *Journal of Psychoactive Drugs* 22(3):333.

Woolley, Sir Leonard. (1953). A Forgotten Kingdom: Being a Record of the Results Obtained from the Excavations of Two Mounds Atchana and Al Mina in the Turkish Hatay. London: Max Parrish.

Wright, M. R. (1981). *Empedocles: The Extant Fragments.* New Haven: Yale University Press.

Yardi, M. R. (Trans.). (1979). *The Yoga of Patanjali.* Poona: Bhandarkar Oriental Research Institute.

Yoke, Ho Peng. (1982). *The Swinging Pendulum: Science in East and West with Special Reference to China.* Hong Kong: University of Hong Kong.

Yule, Henry. (Trans.). (1920). *The Book of Sir Marco Polo.* 3 vols. London: John Murray.

Zaehner, R. C. (1955). *Zurvan: A Zoroastrian Dilemma.* New York: Biblio Tanem.

Zaehner, R. C. (1961). *The Dawn and Twilight of Zoroastrianism.* New York: Putnam's Sons.

Zohar. (n.d.). Translated by Harry Sperling and Maurice Simon. 5 vols. New York: The Rebecca Bennet Publications Inc.

INDEX